The Perioperative Medicine Consult Handbook

D1215081

The Perioperative Medicine Consult Handbook

Second Edition

Molly Blackley Jackson, M.D.
Division of General Internal Medicine, Department of Medicine,
University of Washington Medical Center
Seattle, WA, USA

Somnath Mookherjee, M.D.
Division of General Internal Medicine, Department of Medicine,
University of Washington Medical Center
Seattle, WA, USA

Nason P. Hamlin, M.D., F.A.C.P.
Division of General Internal Medicine, Department of Medicine,
University of Washington Medical Center
Seattle, WA, USA

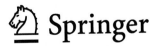 Springer

Editors
Molly Blackley Jackson, M.D.
Division of General Internal
  Medicine
Department of Medicine
University of Washington
  Medical Center
Seattle, WA, USA

Somnath Mookherjee, M.D.
Division of General Internal
  Medicine
Department of Medicine
University of Washington
  Medical Center
Seattle, WA, USA

Nason P. Hamlin, M.D., F.A.C.P.
Division of General Internal
  Medicine
Department of Medicine
University of Washington
  Medical Center
Seattle, WA, USA

ISBN 978-3-319-09365-9   ISBN 978-3-319-09366-6 (eBook)
DOI 10.1007/978-3-319-09366-6
Springer Cham Heidelberg New York Dordrecht London

Library of Congress Control Number: 2014951510

Springer is part of Springer Science+Business Media (www.springer.com)

Dedication

We dedicate this handbook to Chris Wong, for his foundational work on all previous editions.

We also thank the residents and students at the University of Washington, who inspire us to be lifelong teachers and learners.

Preface

The goal of this handbook is to support our colleagues (medical providers, trainees, and students) in providing thoughtful, evidence-based perioperative patient care. In the pages that follow, we aim to provide a focused review of medical issues that arise around the time of surgery along with suggested management strategies based on both the science and art of perioperative medicine.

The foundation of excellence in the care of surgical patients is teamwork. Collaboration and clear communication between the perioperative medicine consultant, surgeon, anesthesiologist, primary and specialty providers, inpatient team (including nurses, pharmacists, therapists, etc.), and the patient improves care, advances the knowledge of each team member, and is incredibly enjoyable. This text was created in partnership with dozens of colleagues at the University of Washington Medical Center, Harborview Medical Center, and the Seattle Veterans Affairs Puget Sound Health Care System. It has been our great privilege to learn and serve our patients together.

Seattle, WA, USA
Molly Blackley Jackson
Somnath Mookherjee
Nason P. Hamlin

Acknowledgments

Amit D. Bhrany, M.D.
Assistant Professor
Department of Otolaryngology
University of Washington
Surgical Procedures Overview

Flavia B. Consens, M.D.
Associate Professor
Department of Neurology
University of Washington
Department of Anesthesiology and Pain Medicine
University of Washington
Obstructive Sleep Apnea and Obesity Hypoventilation Syndrome

Anthony DeSantis, M.D.
Clinical Associate Professor
Division of Metabolism, Endocrinology and Nutrition
Department of Medicine
University of Washington
Diabetes

Cora Espina, M.N., A.R.N.P., C.W.C.N.
Teaching Assistant
Division of Metabolism, Endocrinology and Nutrition
Department of Medicine
University of Washington
Diabetes

Michael F. Fialkow, M.D., M.P.H.
Associate Professor
Department of Obstetrics and Gynecology

University of Washington
Surgical Procedures Overview

Beatrice Franco, R.N., B.S.N., O.C.N.
Clinical Nurse Coordinator
Seattle Cancer Care Alliance
Sickle Cell Disease

Greg Gardner, M.D.
Professor
Division of Rheumatology
Department of Medicine
Adjunct Professor
Department of Orthopaedics and Sports Medicine
Adjunct Professor
Department of Rehabilitation Medicine
University of Washington
Rheumatoid Arthritis, Systemic Lupus Erythematosus, Gout and Pseudogout

Steven Goldberg, M.D.
Clinical Associate Professor
Division of Cardiology
Department of Medicine
University of Washington
Ischemic Heart Disease

John L. Gore, M.D., M.S.
Assistant Professor
Department of Urology
University of Washington
Surgical Procedures Overview

Wei Hao, M.D., Ph.D.
Clinical Associate Professor
Division of Metabolism, Endocrinology and Nutrition
Department of Medicine
University of Washington
Diabetes

Irl B. Hirsch, M.D.
Professor
Division of Metabolism, Endocrinology and Nutrition
Department of Medicine
University of Washington
Diabetes

Reena Julka, M.D.
Attending Physician
Central Dupage Hospital
Venous Thromboembolic Disease, Chronic Kidney Disease, Patients with Solid Organ Transplant

Janet Kelly, Pharm.D.
Clinical Professor
Department of Pharmacy
University of Washington
Diabetes

Saurabh Khandelwal, M.D.
Assistant Professor
Division of General Surgery
Department of Surgery
University of Washington School of Medicine
Bariatric Surgery, Surgical Procedures Overview

Barbara A. Konkle, M.D.
Professor
Division of Hematology
Department of Medicine
University of Washington
Disorders of Hemostasis

Seth Leopold, M.D.
Professor
Department of Orthopaedics and Sports Medicine
University of Washington
Surgical Procedures Overview

Daniel W. Lin, M.D.
Professor
Department of Urology
University of Washington
Surgical Procedures Overview

Iris W. Liou, M.D.
Assistant Professor
Division of Gastroenterology
Department of Medicine
University of Washington
Liver Disease

Frederick A. Matsen, M.D.
Professor
Department of Orthopaedics and Sports Medicine
University of Washington
Surgical Procedures Overview

Suzanne B. Murray, M.D.
Associate Professor
Department of Psychiatry and Behavioral Sciences
University of Washington
Decision-Making Capacity

Ashok Reddy, M.D.
Robert Wood Johnson Foundation Clinical Scholar
Perelman School of Medicine at University of Pennsylvania
Valvular Heart Disease, Chronic Kidney Disease

Cindy Sayre, Ph.D.(c), A.R.N.P.
Associate Administrator, Patient Care Services & Professional Practice
University of Washington Medical Center
Diabetes

Laurie A. Soine, Ph.D., A.R.N.P.
Teaching Associate
Division of Cardiology
Department of Medicine
Teaching Associate
Division of Nuclear Medicine and Cardiology
Department of Radiology
University of Washington
Cardiovascular Risk Stratification

Lauge Sokol-Hessner, M.D.
Assistant Professor
Division of General Medicine and Primary Care
Department of Medicine
Beth Israel Deaconess Medical Center
Postoperative Ileus

Matthew Sweet, M.D.
Assistant Professor
Division of Vascular Surgery
Department of Surgery
University of Washington
Surgical Procedures Overview

Renata R. Urban, M.D.
Assistant Professor
Department of Obstetrics and Gynecology
University of Washington
Surgical Procedures Overview

Gail A. Van Norman, M.D.
Professor
Department of Anesthesiology and Pain Medicine
University of Washington
Decision-Making Capacity

Christopher J. Wong, M.D.
Assistant Professor
Division of General Internal Medicine
Department of Medicine
University of Washington
Beta-Blockers, Atrial Fibrillation, Cerebrovascular Disease, Epilepsy and Seizure Disorders, Venous Thromboembolic Disease, Postoperative Evaluation, Postoperative Fever

Contents

Contributors

Gabrielle Berger, M.D.
Division of General Internal Medicine, Department of Medicine, University of Washington, Seattle, WA, USA

John H. Choe, M.D., M.P.H.
Division of General Internal Medicine, Department of Medicine, University of Washington, Seattle, WA, USA

Paul B. Cornia, M.D.
Division of General Internal Medicine, Department of Medicine, University of Washington, Seattle, WA, USA

Sandra M. Demars, M.D.
Division of General Internal Medicine, Department of Medicine, University of Washington, Seattle, WA, USA

Joana Lima Ferreira, M.D.
Division of General Internal Medicine, Department of Medicine, University of Washington, Seattle, WA, USA

Lindsay Frank, R.D., C.N.S.D.
University of Washington, Seattle, WA, USA

Divya Gollapudi, M.D.
Division of General Internal Medicine, Department of Medicine, University of Washington, Seattle, WA, USA

Anna L. Golob, M.D.
Division of General Internal Medicine, Department of Medicine, University of Washington, Seattle, WA, USA

Nason P. Hamlin, M.D.
Division of General Internal Medicine, Department of Medicine, University of Washington, Seattle, WA, USA

Ronald Huang, M.D., M.P.H.
Division of General Internal Medicine, Department of Medicine, University of Washington, Seattle, WA, USA

Molly Blackley Jackson, M.D.
Division of General Internal Medicine, Department of Medicine, University of Washington, Seattle, WA, USA

Kay M. Johnson, M.D., M.P.H.
Division of General Internal Medicine, Department of Medicine, University of Washington, Seattle, WA, USA

Elizabeth Kaplan, M.D.
Division of General Internal Medicine, Department of Medicine, University of Washington, Seattle, WA, USA

Tyler Lee, M.D.
Division of General Internal Medicine, Department of Medicine, University of Washington, Seattle, WA, USA

Jennifer R. Lyden, M.D.
Division of General Internal Medicine, Department of Medicine, University of Washington, Seattle, WA, USA

Karen A. McDonough, M.D.
Division of General Internal Medicine, Department of Medicine, University of Washington, Seattle, WA, USA

Kara J. Mitchell, M.D.
Division of General Internal Medicine, Department of Medicine, University of Washington, Seattle, WA, USA

Somnath Mookherjee, M.D.
Division of General Internal Medicine, Department of Medicine, University of Washington, Seattle, WA, USA

Brian S. Porter, M.D.
Division of General Internal Medicine, Department of Medicine, University of Washington, Seattle, WA, USA

Ashok Reddy, M.D.
Robert Wood Johnson Foundation, Princeton, NJ, USA
Perelman School of Medicine at University of Pennsylvani,
Seattle, WA, USA

G. Alec Rooke, M.D.
Department of Anesthesiology and Pain Medicine, University
of Washington, Seattle, WA, USA

Christina Ryan, M.D.
Division of General Internal Medicine, Department of
Medicine, University of Washington, Seattle, WA, USA
Department of Neurological Surgery, University of
Washington, Seattle, WA, USA

Nina Saxena, M.D.
Division of General Internal Medicine, Department of
Medicine, University of Washington, Seattle, WA, USA

Sabeena Setia, M.D.
Division of General Internal Medicine, Department of
Medicine, University of Washington, Seattle, WA, USA

Tara Spector, M.D.
Division of General Internal Medicine, Department of
Medicine, University of Washington, Seattle, WA, USA

Rachel E. Thompson, M.D.
Division of General Internal Medicine, Department of
Medicine, University of Washington, Seattle, WA, USA

Gail A. Van Norman, M.D.
Department of Anesthesiology and Pain Medicine, University
of Washington, Seattle, WA, USA

Kelly Wentworth, M.D.
Division of Hospital Medicine, Department of Medicine,
University of California San Francisco, San Francisco, CA,
USA

Andrew A. White, M.D.
Division of General Internal Medicine, Department of
Medicine, University of Washington, Seattle, WA, USA

Christopher J. Wong, M.D.
Division of General Internal Medicine, Department of
Medicine, University of Washington, Seattle, WA, USA

Jeanie C. Yoon, M.D.
Division of General Internal Medicine, Department of
Medicine, University of Washington, Seattle, WA, USA

Chapter 1
Introduction

Kara J. Mitchell and Nason P. Hamlin

Perioperative medicine consultation is an exciting and evolving field. We believe that collaboration between internists, anesthesiologists, and surgeons improves patient care, especially for patients with serious or complex medical conditions. We created this handbook to provide guidance for the general medical care of a patient planning for and recovering from noncardiac surgery. The information presented here is based on a combination of clinical experience, guidelines, and evidence-based medicine.

As with any handbook, the material presented is simply a guide and is no substitute for clinical judgment and individualized patient care.

GENERAL GUIDELINES

PREOPERATIVE ROLE
- Risk-stratify patients prior to surgery (AVOID the term "cleared for surgery")
- Provide recommendations to optimize a patient's condition prior to surgery
- Anticipate perioperative events, and suggest potential ways of mitigating the risk

PERIOPERATIVE ROLE
- Provide postoperative advice with regard to a patient's medical problems
- Identify and manage medical complications of surgery that may arise

M.B. Jackson et al. (eds.), *The Perioperative Medicine Consult Handbook*, DOI 10.1007/978-3-319-09366-6_1, © Springer International Publishing Switzerland 2015

Medicine is medicine, whether a patient has just undergone, or is about to undergo, a surgical procedure. Creating a differential diagnosis, weighing risks and benefits, and providing timely treatment—none of these skills disappear when we see a patient perioperatively. There are, however, a few key characteristics that distinguish postoperative patients:

- Natural history: Most patients should get better if their case is uncomplicated.
- NPO status: Administration of nutrition and/or medications may be restricted for a period of time. Medications may need to be given per rectum, sublingually, intravenously, transdermally, or via inhalation.
- Medication side effects: Most patients receive opioid-type pain medications and are at risk for opioid-related complications: delirium, decreased level of consciousness, respiratory depression, constipation, and urinary retention. Most patients have received sedation and are at risk for aspiration, delirium, and other complications from sedating medications.
- Lines and tubes: Patients may begin their postoperative course with more lines and tubes than medical patients; these are removed as recovery progresses.
- Third spacing: Patients undergoing many types of surgery (especially abdominal surgery) have significant third spacing of fluids and are thus, at least initially, intravascularly volume depleted.

The medical consultant should use caution or refrain from making recommendations about certain subjects, unless first discussed with the patient's surgeon or anesthesiologist (see Table 1.1).

COMMUNICATION IS VITAL!

KEEP UP A DIALOGUE WITH THE SURGICAL TEAM

- Always call with critical recommendations. Do not wait for the surgical team to discover an important recommendation that you made on morning rounds when they make evening rounds.
- Know the habits of your primary surgical team—different surgeons round at different times, and surgery teams have varying compositions of students, house staff, physician assistants, nurse practitioners, and attending physicians.

TABLE 1.1 SUBJECTS TO DISCUSS WITH THE PATIENT'S SURGEON OR ANESTHESIOLOGIST

Avoid recommendations on these subjects	
Type of anesthesia; invasive intraoperative monitoring such as pulmonary artery (PA) catheters or transesophageal echocardiography (TEE)	These decisions are best left to the anesthesiologist
Per rectum (PR) meds in any surgery with bowel manipulation (including abdominal surgery, cystectomy, prostatectomy, and gynecologic surgery)	PR medications may affect the surgical site
Diet advancement with abdominal surgery	Let the surgery team advance the diet

Discuss with the surgical team before making recommendations or writing orders on these subjects	
Venous thromboembolism (VTE) chemoprophylaxis	Good to recommend, but first discuss bleeding risk with the surgery team
Anticoagulation, including antiplatelet agents	Bleeding risk needs to be discussed with the surgery team
Pain medications	Pain medications should be handled by a single team or service to maintain consistency
Transfusion of blood products	If a patient truly requires a transfusion, it is best to discuss with the surgery team first (see Chap. 26)
Antibiotics	The possibility of infection should be discussed with the surgical team; prophylactic antibiotics are generally discontinued within 24 h of surgery. Antibiotic use risks *Clostridium difficile* infection, antibiotic-associated diarrhea, antibiotic resistance, and side effects
Postoperative fever workup, especially within the first 72 h	Early postoperative fever may be due to cytokine release or other causes and not due to infection (see Chap. 45)

- In general, it is acceptable to discuss your recommendations with the patient and family. Be careful, however, when discussing issues specific to the surgery—these are usually best left to the surgeon. There may also be recommendations that are pending your discussion with the surgeon; it is preferable to wait until that discussion has taken place before speaking with the patient and family.

DOCUMENTATION IN THE MEDICAL RECORD IS ESSENTIAL!

It is best to document your recommendations immediately after seeing the patient. You may have communicated very important recommendations verbally—but they must also be in the chart to:
- Make your recommendations official
- Limit risk for confusion or errors when submitting orders
- Improve communication with other providers involved in the patient's care

INITIAL CONSULTS

- Make sure that the name of the provider requesting consultation and reason for consultation is documented in the chart (e.g., "Dr._____ has requested Medicine Consultation for advice regarding management of diabetes.").
- For format of initial consultation, see Chap. 3. Be brief yet thorough and specific.
- Include your contact information.

FOLLOW-UP NOTES

- In general, a note should be completed every day in the chart.
- If you plan to follow the patient less frequently than daily, you should communicate this in the chart: "I will follow up with the patient after surgery" or "Dr._____ will be on call this weekend, but will not plan to see the patient unless you call. Please call if questions arise. I will follow up with the patient on Monday."

- Assessments should be by diagnosis, not organ system: e.g., "diabetes," not "endocrine." Start with the most important medical diagnosis, e.g., "atrial fibrillation," instead of "post-op AAA repair."
- In most cases, you should also communicate with the primary team verbally and document in your note with whom you have spoken.

"COMANAGEMENT" VERSUS "CONSULTATION"

Each hospital and service has a unique balance of comanagement versus consultation. Some surgical services work with internal medicine physicians purely as consultants and ask their advice as needed. In other hospitals, internists actively manage all the medical aspects of a patient's perioperative care, including performing daily assessments, being the first call for nursing staff, and writing orders. See Chap. 2 for further details.

Ultimately, the level of assistance that should be provided depends on your preferences and those of the primary service; clear communication is the key to defining this balance.

Chapter 2
Styles of Medical Consultation

Rachel E. Thompson and Nason P. Hamlin

Medicine departments at many academic institutions have created Medicine Consult Services that provide consultative and perioperative care in the hospital. At some institutions consult services are engaged in both pre- and postoperative care, providing continuity for patients. At other institutions, solely preoperative evaluations and recommendations are provided for surgeons to incorporate into their care. In yet another model, consultations are only available postoperatively. Other models have included comanagement agreements for certain situations, commonly with orthopedic or neurosurgical colleagues.

At the University of Washington Medical Center, where most of the complex surgery is elective, there is a consultative, teaching, and continuity model. The Medicine Consult Service is staffed by internists specializing in perioperative medicine. Comprehensive outpatient medical consultations are done at the request of the surgeon. The same internist who performs the outpatient consultation follows the patient daily when admitted to the hospital for surgery, serving as a consultant (not a comanager). The internist advises and teaches the surgical teams about the medical aspects of perioperative care. New inpatient perioperative consultations are also performed and followed by the Medicine Consult Service physicians. This continuity model minimizes handoffs and enhances satisfaction for patients, surgeons, and the medical consultant.

At Harborview Medical Center, our county hospital run by the University of Washington, there is a smaller, but growing, preoperative practice that was modeled after the University's clinic. The larger practice at present is the inpatient consultative service—this is a teaching service with medical, surgical, and anesthesia residents overseen by an internist who specializes in perioperative care. Harborview is a regional level 1 trauma center and thus many of the

M.B. Jackson et al. (eds.), *The Perioperative Medicine Consult Handbook*, DOI 10.1007/978-3-319-09366-6_2, © Springer International Publishing Switzerland 2015

surgeries are unplanned; medicine consultation is typically requested when surgical patients are identified as medically complex or if medical complications arise postoperatively.

In community hospitals, hospitalists and primary care providers often incorporate perioperative care into their daily work. This can entail caring directly for surgical patients admitted to the hospitalist service but can also mean providing consultation and recommendations to surgical colleagues. Some hospitalist practices have a specified individual available daily for consultations; others perform both primary and consultative care within any given day. Comanagement is also entering into some community practices where a hospitalist may work on a surgical unit or with a particular surgical service. In some cases, preoperative clinics are available which are run by anesthesiologists or in partnership with medical practitioners.

The optimal method of medical consultation is unknown and is likely best tailored to meet the needs of each hospital's patients and care delivery structure. As the field grows, we continue to develop the art and science of best perioperative care practices, improve testing strategies, avoid unnecessary cost, minimize complications, and optimize patient outcomes.

Chapter 3
The Preoperative Evaluation

Molly Blackley Jackson and Christopher J. Wong

BACKGROUND

The "preop" remains a common and important role for the medical consultant. A good preoperative evaluation provides a baseline for the patient's preoperative state, identifies perioperative risks for the patient and surgical team, makes recommendations to help mitigate risk, and serves as a starting point for postoperative management of a patient's medical conditions.

EVALUATION

KEY ELEMENTS OF THE PREOPERATIVE EVALUATION
See Table 3.1 for a summary of key elements of the evaluation and Table 3.2 for suggested preoperative review of systems. Helpful questions to clarify during the initial evaluation include:

What Is the Surgical Risk?
Guidelines from the American Colleges of Cardiology and American Heart Association in 2014 suggest a stepwise approach to assessment of perioperative risk [1]. However, these guidelines do not account for the hundreds of types of surgery in existence, and therefore, one must use clinical judgment to estimate the surgical risk. Additionally, these

M.B. Jackson et al. (eds.), *The Perioperative Medicine Consult Handbook*, DOI 10.1007/978-3-319-09366-6_3,
© Springer International Publishing Switzerland 2015

TABLE 3.1 ELEMENTS OF THE PREOPERATIVE EVALUATION

Requesting physician	Usually the surgeon, sometimes a PCP or specialist, or anesthesiologist
Consult for	Specific reason for or question for consultation
Chief complaint	Include the intended surgical procedure
Date of surgery	(If known)
PCP/active consultants	List here
HPI	A brief summary of the history as it pertains to the proposed surgery. As the surgical workup has already been completed by the surgery team, only the most important elements should be repeated in the medical preoperative HPI
Active and past medical problems	Focus on the ones for which advice has been requested (e.g., diabetes and hypertension) but be complete
Past surgical history and past surgical complications	Especially assess medical complications such as bleeding, thrombosis, infection, delirium, cardiovascular events, and respiratory problems
Drug sensitivities	Include type of reaction(s)
Medications	Include prescription, over-the-counter, and herbal preparations
Family history	Assess family history of problems with anesthesia, or bleeding/clotting disorders, in addition to the standard family history
Social history	Patient's living situation and care network— especially important if there are postop complications requiring additional support after discharge
Habits	Smoking (see Chap. 27) Alcohol (see Chap. 43) Illicit/recreational drugs
Review of systems	See Table 3.2
Functional status and exercise tolerance	Independent, partially dependent, or dependent? Performs own ADLs? Number of blocks able to walk at a normal pace Number of flights of stairs
Physical exam	See chapter text and Table 3.3
Studies	See chapter text and Table 3.4
Assessment	Include • Problem list • Risk assessment, including cardiopulmonary risks
Recommendations	Be specific (doses of drugs, etc.) and concise Include preventative measures, e.g., VTE prophylaxis

TABLE 3.2 PREOPERATIVE REVIEW OF SYSTEMS (ROS)

Constitutional	Fevers, weight change (quantify), chills, night sweats, unexplained falls
Eyes	Visual changes or impairment
Ears/nose/mouth/throat	Sinus pain/pressure, hearing impairment, frequent nose bleeds, tooth pain
Cardiovascular	Chest pain, orthopnea, PND, palpitations, edema, syncope or presyncope, claudication symptoms, history of CHF, CAD, valvular disorder, arrhythmia, murmur, hypertension
Respiratory	Dyspnea (at rest and/or exertion), cough, wheeze, snoring/choking/gasping, witnessed apnea, daytime sleepiness/napping, history of COPD, asthma, OSA, other lung disease
Gastrointestinal	Abdominal pain, difficulty swallowing, nausea/vomiting, diarrhea, constipation, heartburn/reflux, black or bloody bowel movements, abdominal swelling, history of liver disease, peptic ulcer disease, or other gastrointestinal disorders
Genitourinary	Dysuria, hematuria, hesitancy, urgency, urinary retention or incontinence, first day of last menstrual period, contraception use (if relevant), vaginal/penile discharge, history of frequent UTIs, kidney disease
Musculoskeletal	Joint or muscular pain, problems with mobility, history of arthritic or rheumatologic disease
Skin	Rash, wound healing problems, sensitivities (e.g., tapes), skin color changes (jaundice, hyperpigmentation)
Neurologic	Difficulty with balance/speech/memory/cognition, tremor, neuropathy, headache, history of seizures, cerebrovascular disease including TIA or CVA, chronic pain, history of delirium
Psychiatric	Depression, anxiety, psychosis, insomnia
Endocrine	Hot/cold intolerance, fatigue, dry skin, history of diabetes, thyroid disease, recent steroid use, orthostasis, flushing, polydipsia, polyuria
Hematologic	Easy bruising or bleeding, history of anemia, excessive bleeding, use of anticoagulants, personal or family history of hemophilia or thromboembolic disease, blood transfusion preferences
Allergic/immunologic	Environmental allergies, history of significant allergic response (dyspnea, wheezing, swelling, rash) to an exposure, including anaphylaxis

guidelines refer to the risk of cardiovascular complications, not over-all morbidity or mortality. Factors to take into consideration include:

- Duration of general anesthesia (surgery longer than 8 h has been associated with increased risk of complications) [2]
- Emergency surgery (generally considered higher risk)
- Estimated blood loss
- Surgical location and related complications (e.g., abdominal surgery may be more risky in a patient with cirrhosis)

What Are the Patient's Risk Factors?

A thorough medical history will help identify patients at risk for cardiopulmonary complications, bleeding, thrombosis, or increased risk of delirium. The sections in this handbook that follow are useful guides for specific conditions. Consider reading Chaps. 6 and 27 for all patients, and other sections as pertinent.

How Urgent Is the Surgery?

The urgency of surgery is a critical part of the preoperative evaluation. For example, a patient with significant cardiovascular risk might reasonably undergo stress testing for a major elective procedure, but may forego such testing prior to a necessary, urgent surgery for cancer. In the latter case, medical management may be preferred, as a positive preoperative stress test is unlikely to lead to coronary surgery or revascularization prior to the cancer surgery.

PHYSICAL EXAM

The basic preoperative examination should include a comprehensive cardiovascular and pulmonary exam, with other elements of the examination as indicated by the patient's history. The careful examiner should consider diagnoses that are associated with substantial perioperative risk and know the physical examination findings that might support these diagnoses; considerations for an extended preoperative physical exam for select patients is included in Table 3.3. The medicine consultant should be particularly vigilant for evidence of:

- Significant valvular heart disease
- Heart failure with volume overload
- Cardiac arrhythmias
- Pulmonary hypertension
- Liver disease
- Adrenal insufficiency

TABLE 3.3 THE EXTENDED PREOPERATIVE PHYSICAL EXAM

Vital signs	Include blood pressure, resting heart rate, room air oxygen saturation, and weight
General	Describe general appearance
Eyes/ears/nose/mouth/throat	Assess pupillary symmetry and response to light; survey for icterus and conjunctival pallor. Survey for oropharyngeal lesions, discoloration; note dentition
Cardiovascular	Routine inspection and palpation for heaves, thrills, apical impulse. Auscultation with special attention for volume of S1/2, murmurs, gallops. Assess JVP. Assess for peripheral edema
Respiratory	Assess work of breathing, and conduct routine auscultation (for wheeze, rales, rhonchi); assess for increased expiratory time, especially in patients with obstructive lung disease. Assess for Cheyne–Stokes breathing (associated with decreased cardiac ejection fraction), clubbing
Gastrointestinal	Routine inspection (especially for previous surgical scars and distention), palpation, auscultation
Genitourinary	Typically deferred unless indicated by history or reason for surgery
Musculoskeletal	Assess for muscular bulk/tone/symmetry
Hematologic/lymphatic	Survey for pallor, ecchymoses, petechiae. Consider lymph node survey in select patients
Neurologic	Consider basic assessment of orientation and strength. Consider testing memory and cognition in older patients (see Chap. 40). If history of stroke or other intracranial lesion, consider cranial nerve testing, extremity strength and sensory testing, gait, cerebellar examination
Psychiatric	Note affect, speech pace, thought content
Skin	Survey for jaundice, petechiae, ecchymoses, hyperpigmentation, pallor

STUDIES

Best evidence suggests that many common preoperative studies do not need to be ordered routinely (see Table 3.4). Inappropriate preoperative testing may lead to unnecessary delays of surgery. Good communication between the medical consultant, patient, surgeon, and anesthesia team is essential when considering preoperative testing that may affect the timing of surgery.

TABLE 3.4 PREOPERATIVE TESTING

PT, PTT	Not required unless personal or family history of bleeding diathesis
	Obtain PT/INR in patients taking warfarin
CBC	Consider if history or exam suggests abnormality
	Consider hematocrit in older patients undergoing major surgery, or any patient undergoing surgery in which major blood loss is expected
Basic metabolic panel	Consider if history or exam suggests abnormality
	Consider creatinine in older patients undergoing intermediate- or high-risk surgery, or in any patient for whom nephrotoxins will be used, or large fluid shifts or hypotension likely
Liver function tests	Consider only if history or exam suggests abnormality
Urinalysis	Consider only if history or exam suggests abnormality
Pregnancy testing	Consider in all women of reproductive age prior to surgery
ECG	Not useful for asymptomatic patients undergoing low-risk surgery
	Reasonable to obtain in patients with coronary artery disease, significant arrhythmia, peripheral arterial disease, cerebrovascular disease, or structural heart disease (unless undergoing low-risk surgery)
	Consider in patients without above risk factors, but undergoing higher risk surgery [1]
Chest X-ray	As a general rule, not necessary
	May be helpful for patients ≥50 years old undergoing thoracic, upper abdominal, or AAA surgery or who have significant cardiac or respiratory disease [3]
Pulmonary function tests (PFTs)	Obtain only if needed to diagnose previously unknown obstructive lung disease; consider spirometry to assist with risk prediction
	Used in some surgery-specific protocols (e.g., thoracic surgery)
Arterial blood gas (ABG)	Obtain only if suspicion for hypoxemia or CO_2 retention that would affect postop management

ASSESSMENT

SUMMARIZE RISK ASSESSMENT

The preoperative evaluation and recommendations should be summarized in a concise but thorough note. First, state whether the patient is of acceptable risk to undergo surgery. Avoid the term "clearance"—this term implies that nothing will go wrong. There may be complications with any surgical procedure; the key assessment is whether the anticipated benefits outweigh the risks. Next, describe risks in more detail. Consider using risk calculators, especially for the likelihood of cardiac complications, but in general, we recommend avoiding quoting specific percent risk, favoring instead more broad language, e.g., "Mr.___ is at elevated risk for cardiovascular complications due to ...."

Example

"Mr. ____ presents for elective total hip arthroplasty. He is an acceptable candidate for this surgery. He is at increased risk for cardiovascular complications due to diabetes and a prior stroke. However, his exercise tolerance is good; thus, I do not recommend further cardiac testing prior to this procedure. He is at increased risk for pulmonary complications due to emphysema and obstructive sleep apnea. His pulmonary disease remains stable, and his sleep apnea is well treated. Finally, he is at risk for postoperative delirium."

MAKE SPECIFIC RECOMMENDATIONS

Specific recommendations for perioperative management are helpful, including providing suggestions for preoperative testing (if any), guidance on perioperative medication management, management of chronic medical conditions, and thoughtful anticipatory advice to mitigate potential perioperative complications.

Example

Recommendations
1. Proceed with surgery without further cardiac testing.
2. Continue beta-blocker postoperatively. He is anticipated to be taking oral medications immediately postop, so he may be given metoprolol 50 mg PO BID (home dose), holding if $SBP < 110$ or $HR < 60$.
3. For VTE prophylaxis, given our institutional formulary, I recommend enoxaparin 30 mg twice daily for at least 10 days.

4. Postoperative pain should be treated, but psychoactive medications should be minimized to avoid delirium.
5. Attention to pulmonary hygiene postoperatively, including use of incentive spirometry every hour while awake.
6. Continue usual tiotropium inhaler postop, with albuterol nebulizers as needed.
7. Follow up with PCP 2–4 weeks postop.

COMMUNICATE YOUR EVALUATION

Excellent communication is the hallmark of a good medicine consultant. We recommend the following as a minimal standard:

- The patient should be informed of your recommendations.
- The consult note should be copied to the surgeon, the primary care provider, and specialists as appropriate.
- If specific recommendations require early attention, or the case is particularly challenging, the referring surgeon or appropriate designee should be contacted directly.
- The anesthesia team should have access to the consult note on the surgical date.
- The consult note should clearly state how you (or partners when appropriate) may be reached with questions.
- Make sure you know who in your institution will be seeing the patient postop—it may be you, the surgery team alone, or a hospitalist—and make this clear in your note for the inpatient team.

REFERENCES

1. Fleisher LA, Fleischmann KE, Auerbach AD, et al. 2014 ACC/AHA guideline on perioperative cardiovascular evaluation and management of patients undergoing noncardiac surgery: a report of the American College of Cardiology/American Heart Association Task Force on Practice Guidelines. J Am Coll Cardiol. 2014. doi:10.1016/j.jacc.2014.07.944.
2. Reilly DF, McNeely MJ, Doerner D, et al. Self-reported exercise tolerance and the risk of serious perioperative complications. Arch Intern Med. 1999;159:2185–92.
3. Qaseem A, Snow V, Fitterman N, et al. Risk assessment for and strategies to reduce perioperative pulmonary complications for patients undergoing noncardiothoracic surgery: a guideline from the American College of Physicians. Ann Intern Med. 2006;144:575–80.

Chapter 4
Perioperative Medication Management

Anna L. Golob and Tyler Lee

BACKGROUND

The management of a patient's home medication regimen around a surgical procedure is an important component of perioperative medicine. At least half of patients undergoing surgery take routine medications [1]. Clinicians must weigh the risk for a patient's routine medications to cause perioperative harm vs. the risk of stopping the medication with regard to the underlying medical condition. This chapter provides guidance for clinicians in this risk–benefit assessment while acknowledging that there is a general lack of outcomes data about routine medication management in the perioperative setting.

PREOPERATIVE EVALUATION

It is essential to obtain a comprehensive medication list including over-the-counter medications, supplements, inhalers, eye drops, and oral contraceptives, as well as usage, dose, and route (e.g., oral, transdermal, subcutaneous) for all medications. Clinicians should also consider the type of surgery and how it may impact perioperative medication management (prolonged postoperative NPO state, likely to affect liver or kidney function and hence drug clearance, etc.).

M.B. Jackson et al. (eds.), *The Perioperative Medicine Consult Handbook*, DOI 10.1007/978-3-319-09366-6_4,
© Springer International Publishing Switzerland 2015

PERIOPERATIVE MANAGEMENT

PREOPERATIVE

If time permits, it is ideal to stop any medication that may prove harmful perioperatively (e.g., monoamine oxidase [MAO] inhibitors, anticoagulants). Essential medications (e.g., corticosteroids, agents, especially beta-blockers, transplant medications) should be continued without interruption when possible. Exercise judgment on the rest (see tables below for specific recommendations and references). Consider using parenteral or topical forms of essential medications if a patient is NPO. Recommendations for preoperative medication management are shown in Table 4.1.

POSTOPERATIVE

Resume usual outpatient medications as tolerated by patient's ability to take oral medications and current and expected medical indication, with certain exceptions (such as diabetes medications if the patient is not eating—see Chap. 13). Always discuss with the surgeon when restarting antiplatelet agents and anticoagulants (see Chaps. 7 and 18), including nonsteroidal anti-inflammatory drugs (NSAIDs).

Most cardiovascular medications should be continued postoperatively. However, a patient's blood pressure often falls postoperatively (especially if the patient has an epidural), so we suggest writing holding parameters for all vasoactive medications. Dose reduction is frequently necessary for the first 2–3 days. Sequentially add back each vasoactive medication as blood pressure permits.

Following some surgeries, particularly those involving major manipulation of the gastrointestinal tract, the administration of oral medications might be temporarily prohibited. For essential medications, consider using alternate formulations such as intravenous, transdermal, or per rectum if available. In other cases, e.g., after gastric bypass surgery, esophagectomy, or with feeding tubes, medications may need to be crushed for administration. Keep in mind that extended-release formulations cannot be crushed, necessitating a substitution with shorter-acting equivalents. We advise reviewing the medication list with a pharmacist and the surgical team to ensure that appropriate adjustments are made.

See Table 4.2 for recommendations on restarting common outpatient medications.

TABLE 4.1 PREOPERATIVE MEDICATION MANAGEMENT

Drugs to hold for at least 2 weeks preoperatively	Aspirin: Hold for a minimum of 1 week; consider 2 weeks for neuro/spine surgery
	Warning: Must evaluate whether patient has received a cardiac stent (see Chap. 7). Note that some surgeons are comfortable continuing aspirin for certain procedures; communicate with surgeon if desirable to continue aspirin in light of newer data
	MAO inhibitors (see Chap. 26 for Parkinson's disease management, e.g., selegilline, rasagiline)
	Oral central alpha agonists (e.g., methyldopa)
	See "Discussion" for clonidine (if necessary to continue; advise converting this to transdermal form)
	Supplements (e.g., fish oil, garlic, gingko, ginseng, ephedra, oral vitamin E)
	Consider holding
	    Oral contraceptive pills (OCPs) (see "Discussion")
	    Selective estrogen receptor modulators (SERMS) (see "Discussion")
	    Menopausal hormone therapy (MHT) (see "Discussion")
	    SSRIs in orthopedic patients (see "Discussion")
	    Antirheumatic agents (see Chap. 35)

Drugs to hold for 4–5 days preoperatively	P2Y$_{12}$ receptor blockers (clopidogrel, prasugrel, ticagrelor): Hold for a minimum of 5 days. *Warning:* Must evaluate whether patient has received a cardiac stent (see Chap. 7) NSAIDs, selective COX-2 inhibitors (generally hold 4–5 half-lives; depending on the NSAID, this may be more or less than 4–5 days. See "Discussion") Dipyridamole (*Persantine*®). If combined with aspirin (*Aggrenox*®), see above Cilostazol, hold for 5 days Anticoagulants (e.g., warfarin, factor Xa inhibitors, low-molecular-weight heparin, direct thrombin inhibitor (see Chap. 18 and consult anticoagulation clinic if available)

(continued)

TABLE 4.1 (CONTINUED)

Drugs to hold on the morning of surgery	Prandial insulin (see Chap. 13)
	Non-insulin diabetes medications (including injectable hypoglycemic agents (e.g., exenatide) and oral hypoglycemic agents)
	Niacin, gemfibrozil, cholestyramine, and colestipol
	Stimulant medications (e.g., methylphenidate)
	Diuretics (see "Discussion")
	ACE-I/ARBs (see "Discussion")
	Dopamine agonists used for Parkinson's Disease (e.g., bromocriptine, pramipexole, ropinirole; see Chap. 26)
Drugs to give on the morning of surgery. Meds should be taken with a small sip of water only	Most cardiac meds (antiarrhythmics, digoxin, nitrates, beta-blockers)
	Certain antihypertensive medications; see "Discussion" on calcium channel blockers
	Pulmonary medications (e.g., inhalers, nebulizers, oral leukotriene inhibitors, pulmonary hypertension agents)
	Endocrine medications (including thyroid meds and corticosteroids; may need stress dosing—see Chap. 14)
	Most GI medications (e.g., H2 blockers, PPIs)
	Most psychoactive meds (except MAOIs and stimulants); see "Discussion" on SSRIs
	Statins (if taken in the morning)
	Seizure medications
	Gabapentin/pregabalin
	Baclofen (oral and intrathecal) to avoid withdrawal
	Eye drops
	Narcotics (coordinate with anesthesia and primary team)
	Transdermal medications
	Transplant medications (see Chap. 42)
	Immunosuppressives
	Antiretrovirals (check with pharmacist and HIV provider regarding possible drug–anesthesia interactions)

TABLE 4.2 POSTOPERATIVE MEDICATION MANAGEMENT

Drugs to restart as soon as clinically possible	Beta-blockers Antiarrhythmics Statins Nebulizers and inhalers Corticosteroids (discuss with surgical team as needed and see Chap. 14) and thyroid meds Most psychiatric medications Seizure medications Parkinson's medications Immunosuppressives, transplant, and antiretroviral medications (discuss with surgery and transplant teams as needed)
Drugs to restart carefully based on clinical status and discussion with surgical team	Antiplatelet agents Anticoagulants (see Chap. 18) Antihypertensives and diuretics Insulin and non-insulin diabetes medications (see Chap. 13)
Drugs to consider holding postoperatively for several weeks	Oral contraceptive pills (OCPs) (recommend discussion of alternative method of contraception as appropriate) Selective estrogen receptor modulators (SERMs) Menopausal hormone therapy (MHT)

SPECIFIC MEDICINE CONSIDERATIONS

ACE Inhibitors (ACE-Is) and Angiotensin Receptor Blockers (ARBs): The perioperative use of ACE-Is and ARBs has been controversial. A number of relatively small studies have suggested that the use of ACE-Is/ARBs on the morning of surgery may lead to excessive intraoperative hypotension [2]. Based on the updated ACC/AHA and ESC/ESA guidelines, if these agents are used for hypertension we recommend that these agents be held the evening before or the morning of surgery unless the patient is persistently hypertensive with a systolic BP consistently above 180 mmHg. If these agents are used for heart failure and left ventricular dysfunction, consider continuing these agents upon thoughtful discussion with the anesthesiologist, surgeon and cardiologist [3, 4]. Of note, the other situation in which these medications should be held is if renal blood flow will be compromised during the surgical procedure (e.g., some AAA repairs).

Antiplatelet Agents: In high-risk patients (e.g., those with cardiovascular or cerebrovascular disease), it may not be feasible or advisable to stop antiplatelet agents for a prolonged period preoperatively. For patients with cardiac stents, especially if placed recently, there must be a thorough evaluation and discussion regarding the risks of stopping antiplatelet therapy, as acute in-stent thrombosis can be fatal (see Chap. 7). It is best to discuss high-risk cases with the patient's cardiologist or neurologist and the surgical team. In some instances, one or more antiplatelet agents (usually aspirin) should be continued perioperatively without interruption or held for a shorter duration of time (e.g., <1 week) [5, 6].

Beta-Blockers: Abrupt withdrawal of beta-blockers can precipitate rebound tachycardia, hypertension, and angina. If the patient already takes a beta-blocker, it should be continued perioperatively (use IV equivalent if NPO). The initiation of beta-blockade strictly for perioperative reasons is no longer routinely recommended in light of evidence of potential harm in low-risk patients—see Chap. 8 for a more detailed discussion.

Calcium Channel Blockers: Generally safe to continue; consider holding perioperatively if the patient's blood pressure runs low preoperatively. Calcium channel blockers are usually continued if given for rate control for atrial fibrillation.

Clonidine: Abrupt withdrawal may precipitate hypertension and tachycardia. Substitute an equivalent dose transdermal patch if possible. It takes 2–3 days for the patches to begin working. If possible, initiate the patch preoperatively. Have the patient take his/her full oral dose on the first day the patch is applied, 1/2 the usual dose on day 2, 1/4 of the usual dose on day 3, then stop the oral medication. Patches are changed every 7 days.

Diuretics: Conventional practice and our recommendation is to hold diuretics on the morning of surgery due to concern for intraoperative hypotension. One small 2010 study, however, found no difference in intraoperative hypotension in a lower-risk patient population [7]. Many patients are intravascularly depleted postoperatively due to third spacing, poor PO intake, etc.; however, some may become hypervolemic from intraoperative resuscitation or maintenance IV fluids, especially in the setting of congestive heart failure (CHF) or chronic kidney disease (CKD).

Statins: Data from a few studies in vascular surgery patients suggest that the use of the HMG-CoA reductase inhibitors (statins) perioperatively may reduce the risk of perioperative cardiovascular events (e.g., MI, angina, stroke) [8, 9]. A recent systemic review suggests treating statin-naïve patients perioperatively may reduce the risk of perioperative atrial fibrillation and myocardial infarction and decrease mean length of hospital stay in both cardiac and noncardiac surgery [10]. For statin-naïve patients, consider initiating a statin prior to vascular surgery and in patients with increased risk for cardiovascular events, as these patients usually also have indications for lipid lowering therapy. If the patient is already on a statin, it should be continued preoperatively and resumed postoperatively when able. These recommendations are consistent with the recently updated ACC/AHA and ESC/ESA guidelines [3, 4].

Oral Contraceptive Pills (OCPs): Increase the risk of thrombosis, especially for high-risk procedures (e.g., hip and knee arthroplasty). Consider stopping 4 weeks preoperatively for moderate- and high-risk procedures; one must weigh the risk of venous thromboembolic event (VTE) against the risk of undesired pregnancy. Recommend discussion of alternative methods of contraception.

Menopausal Hormone Therapy (MHT): Increases the risk of thrombosis, especially for high-risk procedures. If possible, should be discontinued at least 4–6 weeks preoperatively for procedures of moderate or high risk of VTE.

Selective Estrogen Receptor Modulators: Increase the risk of thrombosis, especially for high-risk procedures. If the indication for selective estrogen receptor modulator (SERM) use is breast cancer prevention or osteoporosis, consider stopping 4 weeks preoperatively for procedures that are moderate or high risk for VTE. If the indication for SERM use is breast cancer treatment, discuss risks/benefits of stopping with the patient's oncologist.

Selective Serotonin Reuptake Inhibitors: The putative mechanism for potential increased bleeding risk is an effect on platelet aggregation. A retrospective study from 2003 showed that exposure to serotonergic antidepressants (not necessarily selective) increased the degree of intraoperative bleeding and increased risk of blood transfusion in patients undergoing orthopedic surgery [11]. Interestingly, the transfusion group also had lower baseline hemoglobin values. However, two retrospective cohort studies of patients receiving coronary artery bypass graft surgery did not show a difference in perioperative bleeding or mortality but did show an increase in the volume of red blood cell unit transfusion in the postoperative period among patients on selective serotonin reuptake inhibitors (SSRIs) [12, 13]. A recent retrospective study using administrative data consisting of more 500,000 patients found an association of higher adjusted odds ratio for in-hospital mortality, bleeding, and 30-day readmission rate in patients receiving SSRIs prior to major surgery. Of note, the increased risk for mortality is absent if adjusted for patients with depression [14]. Currently, there is no compelling evidence to recommend the routine discontinuation of SSRIs preoperatively especially in patients being treated for depression. One may consider discontinuing SSRIs prior to major orthopedic surgery based on the surgeon's preferences. If an SSRI is to be discontinued, it should be tapered to avoid withdrawal symptoms.

Monoamine Oxidase Inhibitors and Carbidopa–Levodopa: See Chap. 26.

Nonsteroidal Anti-inflammatory Drugs: NSAIDs vary greatly in half-life, COX-2 selectivity, brand names, and formulations. In general, NSAIDs with shorter half-lives include ibuprofen, indomethacin, diclofenac, and ketoprofen; NSAIDs with longer half-lives include naproxen, nabumetone, meloxicam, and piroxicam. Keep in mind that there are also extended-release preparations of several of the shorter-acting medications.

Opioid Pain Medications: Management of chronic opioid pain medications perioperatively requires discussion with the surgeon, the physician prescribing the pain medications (if different from the surgeon), and the patient. There is limited evidence that patients undergoing orthopedic surgery may have worse outcomes if receiving chronic opioid therapy [15], but whether reduction in preoperative opioid medication results in better outcomes is unknown. Pain management specialist consultation, if available, should be considered for patients receiving chronically high doses of opioid medications preoperatively.

REFERENCES

1. Kennedy JM, van Rij AM, Spears GF, et al. Polypharmacy in a general surgical unit and consequences of drug withdrawal. Br J Clin Pharmacol. 2000;49:353.
2. Comfere T, Sprung J, Kumar MM, et al. Angiotensin system inhibitors in a general surgery population. Anesth Analg. 2005;100:636–44.
3. Fleisher LA, Fleischmann KE, Auerbach AD, Barnason SA, et al. 2014 ACC/AHA guideline on perioperative cardiovascular evaluation and management of patients undergoing noncardiac surgery. J Am Coll Cardiol. 2014. doi:10.1016/j.jacc.2014.07.944.
4. Kristensen SD, Knuuti J, Saraste A, et al. ESC/ESA Guidelines on non-cardiac surgery: cardiovascular assessment and management: The Joint Task Force on non-cardiac surgery: cardiovascular assessment and management of the European Society of Cardiology (ESC) and the European Society of Anaesthesiology (ESA). Eur Heart J. 2014. doi:10.1093/eurheartj/ehu282.
5. Gerstein NS, Schulman PM, Gerstein WH, et al. Should more patients continue aspirin therapy perioperatively? Clinical impact of aspirin withdrawal syndrome. Ann Surg. 2012;255(5):811–9.

6. Peterfreund, RA. Take an aspirin and I'll (safely) put you on-call to the OR in the morning. APSF Newsletter. Spring-Summer 2012
7. Khan NA, Campbell NR, Frost SD, et al. Risk of intraoperative hypotension with loop diuretics: a randomized controlled trial. Am J Med. 2010;123:1059e1–8.
8. Durazzo AE, Machado FS, Ikeoka DT, et al. Reduction in cardiovascular events after vascular surgery with atorvastatin: a randomized trial. J Vasc Surg. 2004;39:967–76.
9. Schouten O, Boersma E, Hoeks SE, et al. Fluvastatin and perioperative events in patients undergoing vascular surgery. N Engl J Med. 2009;361:980–9.
10. Chopra V, Wesorick DH, Sussman JB, et al. Effect of perioperative statins on death, myocardial infarction, atrial fibrillation, and length of stay. Arch Surg. 2012;147(2):181–9.
11. Movig KL, Janssen MW, de Waal MJ. Relationship of serotonergic antidepressants and need for blood transfusion in orthopedic surgical patients. Arch Intern Med. 2003;163:2354–8.
12. Andreasen JJ, Riis A, Hjortdal VE, et al. Effect of selective serotonin reuptake inhibitors on requirement for allogeneic red blood cell transfusion following coronary artery bypass surgery. Am J Cardiovasc Drugs. 2006;6:243–50.
13. Xiong GL, Jiang W, Clare RM, et al. Safety of selective serotonin reuptake inhibitor use prior to coronary artery bypass grafting. Clin Cardiol. 2010;33(6):E94–8.
14. Auerbach AD, Vittinghoff E, Maselli J, et al. Perioperative use of selective serotonin reuptake inhibitors and risks for adverse outcomes of surgery. JAMA Intern Med. 2013;173(12):10751081.
15. Zywel MG, Stroh A, Lee SY, Bonutti PM, Mont MA. Chronic opioid use prior to total knee arthroplasty. J Bone Joint Surg Am. 2011;93:1988–93.

Chapter 5
Anesthesia Pearls

Gail A. Van Norman

BACKGROUND

The anesthesiologist fulfills several critical roles in the perioperative period apart from the actual administration of the anesthetic. The anesthesiologist functions also as a "primary care" physician for the patient's medical conditions in the operating room. Anesthesiologists have a wide range of core medical knowledge as well as broad experience in managing coexisting disease in the operating room. They also have specialty knowledge in cardiovascular and respiratory physiology, and critical event management. Many issues of interest to the anesthesiologist in the perioperative period overlap with concerns of the medicine consultant.

PERIOPERATIVE MANAGEMENT

A primary focus of anesthesia practice is risk management and patient safety. In the preoperative period, some examples of issues that anesthesiologists focus on include the following:

- Relative risk of the surgery in question.
- Current medical comorbidities and whether they have been optimized.
- History or physical exam indications of any undiagnosed medical conditions that could affect anesthesia and surgery.
- What anesthetic techniques are options for surgery, and which best address the medical comorbidities of the patient while providing good surgical conditions.

M.B. Jackson et al. (eds.), *The Perioperative Medicine Consult Handbook*, DOI 10.1007/978-3-319-09366-6_5,
© Springer International Publishing Switzerland 2015

- In what ways physical aspects of the surgery (positioning, site of incision, duration, need for muscle relaxation) affect anesthetic choices and monitoring patients.
- The monitoring (including hemodynamic and neuromuscular monitoring) that is appropriate for the surgery and will mitigate risk.
- Postoperative management of pain, respiratory changes, nausea, and vomiting.
- Discharge issues, such as how soon the patients can be discharged, where the patient will be discharged to, and in whose company.

PEARLS TO CONSIDER

Evidence-based guidelines on anesthesia and surgery are extremely helpful in most cases, but are not always completely applicable, because they fail to account for local differences in surgical practice, as well as important differences among individual surgeons. Issues that can affect whether further workup of a medical condition, or other management, is needed in the perioperative period and are often overlooked include the following:

- *Positioning during surgery*. Some surgeries require sitting position (shoulder, breast, and some neurosurgery). Further cardiac or neurovascular workup may be indicated if the patient will undergo unusual positioning with adverse hemodynamic consequences.
- *Blood loss*. While surgeries can be categorized into major, minor, and minimal blood loss, this is highly dependent on the surgeon, whether the surgery is a revision of a previous one, and the surgical technique. For example, blood loss during spine surgery can range from minor (1–2 unit loss not requiring transfusion) to major/disastrous (up to or exceeding a patient's entire blood volume). Consultation with an anesthesiologist may be helpful in defining these risks for the patient, based both on the surgery and the surgeon performing it.
- *Duration of surgery*. Not all surgeons work alike. One surgeon may routinely finish a lumbar laminectomy in 20 min, for example, while another takes 3 h. Duration of surgery affects anesthetic choices, risks, and perioperative planning. Discussion with the anesthesiologist may facilitate your plans, particularly in high-risk patients.

- *Device management.* All implantable cardiac electronic devices should be interrogated to determine if they either should be turned off or reprogrammed for the operating room during elective surgery. Depending on the institution, this may be done in a preanesthesia clinic or in the preoperative holding area, by a member of either the cardiology or the anesthesiology department (see Chap. 12).
- *Deep brain stimulators.* Devastating central nervous system injuries have been reported in Parkinson's patients with deep brain stimulators, as a result of deep brain electrical injury. The patients should always bring their programmer with them to surgery, at which time these devices will be temporarily turned off. Consultation with the anesthesiologist can help determine if an exception to this general rule can be made.
- *Open vs. laparoscopic surgery.* Although laparoscopic surgery is considered less invasive, physiologic changes during laparoscopy can have serious hemodynamic consequences. Patients may be positioned in extreme upright or extreme Trendelenburg position. Insufflation of the abdomen affects right heart filling. Absorption of CO_2 leads to obligatory hypercapnia. Ventilation is impeded due to high abdominal pressures. For patients who cannot tolerate these changes, other surgical approaches might be appropriate, even if more "invasive."
- *Regional anesthesia is no safer than general anesthesia* for most procedures, with some very limited exceptions. The decision for regional vs. general anesthesia is made based primarily on patient, anesthesiologist, and surgeon preference and postoperative pain management issues. Please consult the anesthesiologist if you have questions.

MEDICINE CONSULT NOTES

For patients with comorbidities that require multidisciplinary support perioperatively, anesthesia teams find the following information helpful in medicine consult notes:

- A list of medical comorbidities and assessment of the current status of each.
- Plans for any further workup or intervention for comorbidities.
- Plans regarding anticoagulation, including timing and medications to be discontinued, and plans for bridging therapy, if any.

- Requests for anything that might be helpful to your postoperative management. For example, you might want central line access, but such access is not needed for the anesthetic per se. The anesthesiologist may be willing to place these lines or others for you while the patient is anesthetized. Please do indicate that you are requesting the line for postoperative issues.

Avoid the following statements or advice for anesthesia teams in medicine consultation notes:

- "Avoid hypoxemia and hypotension," or "watch the patient's hemodynamics" during surgery (or similar statements). Anesthesiologists specialize in understanding the hemodynamic, respiratory, and metabolic changes brought about by the surgery and anesthetic, and how to treat them.
- Instructions about what monitors to use intraoperatively. Anesthesiologists specialize in understanding when the information from a particular monitor (e.g., pulmonary artery catheter) is helpful or not. Statements advising the use of these devices create legal problems when the anesthesiologist's expert opinion differs from yours. Please make any advisory statements that you feel compelled to make flexible enough to accommodate dissent. For example, "consider pulmonary artery catheter."
- Demand a specialist anesthesiologist or make statements that the patient requires them (see below for guidelines). This also creates legal issues if there is disagreement with the specialist. Statements such as "consider cardiac anesthesia" are much more acceptable.
- Recommendations for a specific anesthetic. The anesthesiologist is the specialist best qualified to determine the appropriate and safest anesthetic techniques.

WHEN TO CONSIDER INVOLVING SUBSPECIALTY ANESTHESIOLOGIST

PAIN SPECIALIST

- Patient has medical comorbidities or complex pain issues that will require special techniques.
- Risk factors for postoperative pain management issues include sleep apnea, chronic sedative or opioid use, history of

poor postoperative pain control, history of substance abuse (including alcohol), complex surgery, or history of opioid allergies.

CARDIAC ANESTHESIOLOGIST

- Procedure will involve cardiopulmonary bypass; transesophageal monitoring may be needed.
- Patient has complex congenital heart disease.
- Patient has severe pulmonary hypertension (PA systolic >55 mmHg, particularly if accompanied by right ventricular dysfunction or dilation), pulmonary hypertension accompanied by other cardiac issues (e.g., abnormal left ventricular function, critical coronary disease, associated valvular dysfunction).
- Patients with severe valvular stenosis (due to high likelihood of requiring transesophageal echocardiography monitoring).

OBSTETRICAL ANESTHESIOLOGIST

- Patient is undergoing a complex surgery and is pregnant.

ANESTHESIOLOGY TERMINOLOGY

AMERICAN SOCIETY OF ANESTHESIOLOGISTS CLASS [1]

- I—Healthy
- II—Mild systemic disease
- III—Severe systemic disease
- IV—Severe systemic disease that is a constant threat to life
- V—Moribund, not expected to survive without the operation

This classification system has been shown to be predictive of perioperative complications and mortality. For example, one study showed mortality rates of 0.1, 0.7, 3.5, and 18.3 % for American Society of Anesthesiologists (ASA) class I, II, III, and IV, respectively [2].

MALLAMPATI CLASS

- Refers to the accessibility of the oral airway as seen by the patient opening his or her mouth while seated
- Ranges from class I (can see back of throat, uvula, etc.) to class IV (can only see hard palate)

REFERENCES

1. ASA website. http://www.asahq.org/clinical/physicalstatus.htm. Accessed April 2014.
2. Wolters U, Wolf T, Stutzer H, et al. ASA classification and perioperative variables as predictors of postoperative outcome. Br J Anaesth. 1996;77:217–22.

Chapter 6
Cardiovascular Risk Stratification

Molly Blackley Jackson

BACKGROUND

Perioperative cardiovascular complications pose serious risk to patients, especially those with underlying cardiac disease. The degree of risk varies widely depending on medical comorbidities and type of surgery. A careful medical evaluation before surgery can help inform a discussion of risk for patients and providers and suggest management to mitigate risk.

PREOPERATIVE EVALUATION

A focused history and physical examination (including an assessment of functional capacity) and an understanding of the proposed surgery provide the initial foundation for a discussion of perioperative cardiac risk and can help inform the need for additional evaluation. Guidelines from the American College of Cardiology/American Heart Association (ACC/AHA) and European Societies of Cardiology and Anaesthesiology (ESC/ESA) published in 2014 suggest approaches to perioperative cardiovascular risk stratification that leave some discretion to the provider and patient regarding noninvasive stress testing [1, 2]. We advocate for a similar stepwise approach (Fig. 6.1), while keeping in mind that patients are individuals and guidelines should not be interpreted as strict rules.

The type of surgery, expected blood loss, duration of anesthesia, and anticipated fluid shifts each contribute to surgical stress. Surgical approaches in the same general category may have a broad range of risk (e.g., among intraperitoneal surgeries, the laparoscopic band

M.B. Jackson et al. (eds.), *The Perioperative Medicine Consult Handbook*, DOI 10.1007/978-3-319-09366-6_6,
© Springer International Publishing Switzerland 2015

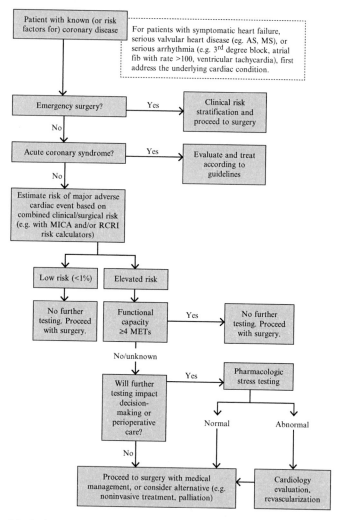

Fig. 6.1 Perioperative Assessment for Coronary Artery Disease. Adapted with permission from [2]

surgery likely has lower risk than a complex open abdominal surgery). Procedures with prolonged anesthesia (especially >8 h) and cases with extensive fluid shifts or blood loss are higher risk for perioperative complications.

TABLE 6.1 EXAMPLES OF ESTIMATED METABOLIC EQUIVALENTS

METs	Activity
1–3	Care of self (eating, dressing, using toilet)
4	Climbing a flight of stairs, walking up a hill, walking on level ground at 4 mph
6	Moderate recreational activity, e.g., dancing, doubles tennis, moderate cycling

Adapted with permission from [3] (Table 10)

FUNCTIONAL CAPACITY/EXERCISE TOLERANCE

Clarifying an individual patient's functional capacity is critical to estimating surgical risk and to decision-making regarding further evaluation. A metabolic equivalent (MET) is a measure of degree of oxygen uptake of sitting at rest and has been used in many studies to help assess functional capacity (Table 6.1) [3]. Patients who are able to achieve four METs without limiting cardiopulmonary symptoms can usually proceed to surgery without further cardiac evaluation. Self-reported reduced exercise tolerance (inability to walk four blocks or climb two flights of stairs) predicts perioperative complications [4].

ESTIMATION OF CARDIAC RISK

There are several clinical tools to estimate perioperative cardiovascular risk, though none have ideal predictive performance. These tools are helpful when used in combination with a traditional medical evaluation and clinical gestalt. When documenting and discussing risk with patients, avoid quoting exact percentage estimates from these tools; rather, indicating that a patient is at low, moderate, or high risk for cardiac complications is more useful (and accurate). Keep in mind that the specific cardiac complications predicted by these tools may be different. Two commonly used calculators include:

MICA / Gupta Perioperative Cardiac Risk Calculator

The MICA (perioperative myocardial infarction or cardiac arrest) risk calculator was created using the American College of Surgeons' 2007 National Surgical Quality Improvement Program (NSQIP) database and evaluated over 200,000 surgical patients for perioperative cardiac complications [5]. The risk model was then validated, and the predictive performance surpassed the commonly used Revised Cardiac Risk Index (RCRI) risk calculator (below). Five major predictors for perioperative myocardial infarct or cardiac arrest were determined: type of surgery, functional status, American Society of

TABLE 6.2 REVISED CARDIAC RISK INDEX

Risk factors (1 pt for each)	# Of risk factors	Risk class	% Major cardiac complications (95 % confidence interval)
■ "High-risk" surgery	0	I	0.4 (0.05–1.5)
– Intraperitoneal	1	II	0.9 (0.3–2.1)
– Intrathoracic	2	III	6.6 (3.9–10.3)
– Suprainguinal vascular	3 or more	IV	11 (5.8–18.4)
■ History of myocardial ischemia (pathologic Q's, angina, nitrates, prior MI, positive stress test)			
■ History of heart failure			Major cardiac complications = MI,
■ History of CVA or TIA			pulmonary edema, cardiac arrest,
■ Preoperative insulin use			complete heart block
Creatinine > 2.0			

Reprinted with permission from [6]

Anesthesiologists class, elevated creatinine, and advanced age. The online calculator is available at: http://www.surgicalriskcalculator.com/miorcardiacarrest.

Revised Cardiac Risk Index

The Revised Cardiac Risk Index (Table 6.2) is an older, well-validated, and easy to use tool, though it may overstate risk in part because anesthesia and surgical techniques have improved since its publication [6]. Patients in the study were 50 years or older and underwent major noncardiac surgery. Note that the RCRI estimates risk of pulmonary edema and heart block, in addition to MI and cardiac arrest.

PREOPERATIVE CARDIAC TESTING

ACC/AHA guidelines recommend the following preoperatively:

12-Lead Electrocardiogram

- Do not obtain routine electrocardiogram (ECG) in asymptomatic patients undergoing low-risk surgical procedures.
- It is reasonable to obtain an ECG (within 3 months of surgery) for patients with known coronary artery disease, significant arrhythmia, peripheral arterial disease, cerebrovascular disease, or significant structural heart disease, except for those undergoing low-risk surgery.

- Consider ECG in patients without above conditions, but undergoing higher risk surgery.
- ACC/AHA guidelines do not support routine ECG based on advanced age alone. However, we consider an ECG in patients age 70 and older in some clinical situations, because finding an abnormality may change our prediction of risk, and will provide a baseline to help interpret changes postoperatively, should the patient develop cardiac complications.

Resting Echocardiography
- Consider transthoracic echo in patients with dyspnea of unknown etiology, or in patients with heart failure and increased dyspnea

CARDIAC STRESS TESTING
Before ordering a stress test, ask yourself: How will the results change my management? What will I do with the data? The goals of stress testing are to risk stratify prior to surgery and to identify patients in whom cardiology consultation, revascularization, or other means of potentially lowering cardiac risk is warranted. If you elect to proceed with noninvasive cardiovascular stress testing, there are several options:

Exercise Testing
The Exercise Tolerance Test (ETT) is a relatively inexpensive and well-validated study to assess functional capacity and symptoms, hemodynamic response to exercise and recovery, and ECG evidence of ischemia. Each of these factors has independent prognostic predictive value.

- The Duke Treadmill Score (DTS) provides a risk score based upon exercise duration on a Standard Bruce Protocol, symptoms, and ST changes [7].
- An ETT study with ECG monitoring coupled with either myocardial perfusion imaging (see below) or transthoracic echocardiography (TTE) can elucidate high-risk features such as a large region of anterior wall ischemia or multiple regions of myocardial infarction that may change perioperative management.
- However, exercise testing is often not possible (e.g., patients with orthopedic limitations, vascular claudication) or not recommended (e.g., patients with large aortic aneurysms).

Pharmacologic Stress Tests
These tests are useful for patients who are unable to exercise adequately. They are thought to have very good negative predictive value (if negative, likelihood of cardiac event is very low), but less good

positive predictive value (if positive, still a weak predictor of perioperative cardiac complications). There are two commonly ordered categories of pharmacologic stress studies:

Dobutamine Stress Echo

- Dobutamine stress echos (DSEs) provide important prognostic information including left/right ventricular size and function, resting wall motion abnormalities consistent with prior infarction, stress-induced wall motion abnormalities suggestive of ischemia, and valvular abnormalities.
- Beta-blockers must be held for 12–24 h prior to study.
- A history of unstable angina, recent MI, ventricular arrhythmias, and severe hypertension are contraindications to high-dose dobutamine infusion.

Vasodilator Myocardial Perfusion Imaging

- Myocardial perfusion imaging (MPI) provides useful prognostic information including left ventricular size and function, fixed perfusion abnormalities consistent with myocardial infarction, and reversible abnormalities consistent with ischemia; the location, extent, and severity of ischemia and/or infarction are reported.
- Single-photon emission computed tomography (SPECT) remains the most commonly utilized imaging modality in nuclear medicine. Positron emission tomography (PET) is less widely available and somewhat more expensive, but offers better image quality (and thus higher sensitivity for ischemia) in patients with morbid obesity, multivessel coronary disease, and/or severe ischemic cardiomyopathy. Likewise, a complete rest/stress perfusion PET can be accomplished in <1 h, with only half the radiation exposure of SPECT.
- A history of either severe aortic stenosis or severe bronchospasm is a contraindication for vasodilator (regadenoson) infusion. However, regadenoson is safe in patients with severe COPD or pulmonary fibrosis.

INTERPRETATION OF STRESS TESTS

ACC/AHA guidelines recommend cardiology evaluation and coronary angiography for patients with the features shown in Table 6.3 on cardiac testing, even if asymptomatic (note that this does not address the issue of preoperative evaluation, rather any patient with these findings regardless of planned surgery) [2]. Even among patients with known cardiac disease, it remains uncertain who should receive

TABLE 6.3 HIGH-RISK NONINVASIVE TEST RESULTS

Resting LVEF <35 %

High-risk treadmill score of ≤ −11

Exercise LVEF <35 %

Stress-induced large perfusion defect (particularly if anterior)

Stress-induced moderate-size multiple perfusion defects

Large, fixed perfusion defect with LV dilatation or increased lung uptake

Stress-induced moderate-size perfusion defect with LV dilatation or increased lung uptake

Wall motion abnormality on stress echo (>2 segments) at low dose of dobutamine or at a low HR (<120 bpm)

Stress echo with extensive ischemia

Reprinted with permission from [8]

revascularization versus medical management alone prior to surgery. ACC/AHA guidelines recommend consideration for revascularization prior to elective surgery in patients with stable angina with significant lesions (especially left main) and patients with unstable cardiac disease. The Coronary Artery Revascularization Prophylaxis (CARP) trial suggested that among patients undergoing elective vascular surgery, elective revascularization (PCI or CABG) does not decrease perioperative mortality, MI, or stroke [9]. However, this trial excluded patients with ≥ 50 % stenosis of the left main coronary artery, left ventricular ejection fraction of less than 20 %, and severe aortic stenosis.

Our practice is to clarify the urgency (and necessity) of the surgery, consider if the patient has an indication for revascularization regardless of surgery, and engage in a discussion of benefits and risks with the patient, surgeon, and cardiologist.

CASE DISCUSSIONS

1. A 55-year-old woman with hypertension and hyperlipidemia is diagnosed with colon cancer. She has no cardiac symptoms but her exercise tolerance is poor. A vasodilator stress MPI scan is positive for a small region of ischemia involving the inferior wall.

   Comment: This patient is undergoing a necessary surgery, which should not be delayed for a low-risk stress test result. Optimum management includes control of hypertension and hyperlipidemia and perioperative attention to pain control, blood pressure control, and signs of ischemia.

2. A 65-year-old man with history of tobacco use, type 2 diabetes mellitus, and poor exercise tolerance is diagnosed with a 5.6 cm abdominal aortic aneurysm (AAA). He has exertional dyspnea. A vasodilator stress MPI scan revealed several areas of ischemia (multiple territories at risk), including a large region of severe myocardial ischemia involving the anterior wall.
   Comment: This patient is considering major elective vascular surgery. He has a high-risk stress test and is likely symptomatic. Surgery should be postponed; cardiology consultation should be initiated. Cardiac catheterization confirmed three-vessel disease with a normal left main. He meets the criteria for CABG regardless of his intended operation and elects to have this done prior to his AAA repair. However, revascularization may not necessarily alter the perioperative outcome.

3. A 60-year-old woman with hypertension, type 2 diabetes mellitus, hyperlipidemia, and chronic obstructive pulmonary disease (COPD) is to undergo partial lobectomy for non-small cell lung cancer. Her exercise tolerance is <4 METs. Vasodilator stress MPI scan is positive for a large area of moderate myocardial ischemia involving the entire anterior wall (LAD distribution).
   Comment: This patient is undergoing thoracic surgery and has significant risk factors for coronary artery disease. Consultation with cardiology including possible cardiac catheterization would be prudent. Several options exist, including:
   (a) Placement of a bare metal stent and postponing surgery for 1 month, if delay would not pose significant risk of spread of cancer
   (b) CABG, single vessel, with combined partial lobectomy
   (c) No intervention based on extrapolating the CARP trial results to nonvascular surgery. Optimize medical management; alert anesthesia
   (d) Defer surgical intervention completely

4. The same patient as in #3 is to undergo elective total knee arthroplasty (TKA) for degenerative joint disease.
   Comment: This patient is undergoing an elective surgery but has a high risk of cardiac complications. Surgery should be delayed and outpatient cardiology evaluation completed.

REFERENCES

1. Kristensen SD, Knuuti J, Saraste A, et al. ESC/ESA Guidelines on non-cardiac surgery: cardiovascular assessment and management: The Joint Task Force on non-cardiac surgery: cardiovascular assessment and management of the European Society of Cardiology (ESC) and the European Society of Anaesthesiology (ESA). Eur Heart J. 2014. doi: 10.1093/eurheartj/ehu282.
2. Fleisher LA, Fleischmann KE, Auerbach AD, et al. 2014 ACC/AHA Guideline on Perioperative Cardiovascular Evaluation and Management of Patients Undergoing Noncardiac Surgery, Journal of the American College of Cardiology (2014), doi: 10.1016/j.jacc.2014.07.944.
3. Fletcher GF, Balady G, Froelicher VF, et al. Exercise standards. A statement for healthcare professionals from the American Heart Association. Circulation. 1995;91:580–615.
4. Reilly DF, McNeely MJ, Doerner D, et al. Self-reported exercise tolerance and the risk of serious perioperative complications. Arch Intern Med. 1999;159:2185–92.
5. Gupta PK, Gupta H, Sundaram A, et al. Development and validation of a risk calculator for prediction of cardiac risk after surgery. Circulation. 2011;124:381–7.
6. Lee TH, Marcantonio ER, Mangione CM, et al. Derivation and prospective validation of a simple index for prediction of cardiac risk of major noncardiac surgery. Circulation. 1999; 100:1043–9.
7. Mark DB, Shaw L, Harrell FE, et al. Prognostic value of a treadmill exercise score in outpatients with suspected coronary artery disease. N Engl J Med. 1991;325:849–53.
8. Scanlon PJ, Faxon DP, Audet AM, et al. ACC/AHA guidelines for coronary angiography: executive summary and recommendations. Circulation. 1999;99:2345–57.
9. McFalls EO, Ward HB, Moritz TE, et al. Coronary-artery revascularization before elective major vascular surgery. N Engl J Med. 2004;351:2795–804.

Chapter 7
Ischemic Heart Disease

Molly Blackley Jackson

BACKGROUND

History of ischemic heart disease is a significant risk factor for perioperative cardiac complications, including postoperative myocardial infarction, heart failure, arrhythmia, cardiac arrest, and death [1]. A careful history and physical exam in patients with ischemic heart disease, including prior infarction and/or extent of coronary artery disease (CAD), is crucial prior to surgery to better assess and communicate risk to the patient and surgeon and to suggest management that may mitigate risk perioperatively.

PREOPERATIVE EVALUATION

HISTORY AND PHYSICAL EXAMINATION
Key historical elements to gather are summarized in Table 7.1. For preoperative cardiac risk assessment and consideration for stress testing, see Chap. 6. Other considerations include:

- Consider electrocardiogram (ECG) in preoperative patients with known CAD, except for those undergoing low-risk surgery. New and/or concerning changes (e.g., pathologic Q wave, ST-T wave changes, or new arrhythmia) may help with risk assessment and/or perioperative optimization. ECG within 90 days of surgical date is generally acceptable [2].
- If symptoms of active cardiac disease (exertional chest pain, dyspnea, recent syncope, etc), consider prompt cardiology evaluation.

M.B. Jackson et al. (eds.), *The Perioperative Medicine Consult Handbook*, DOI 10.1007/978-3-319-09366-6_7,
© Springer International Publishing Switzerland 2015

TABLE 7.1 PREOPERATIVE HISTORY FOR PATIENTS WITH ISCHEMIC HEART DISEASE

History of myocardial ischemia (MI)	Date, symptoms
History of stent placement	Date(s) and (arterial) location of stents Reason for stent (MI? abnormal stress test?) Type of stent: bare metal, drug eluting
History of bypass	Date, vessels bypassed (and harvested)
Current symptoms	Angina, dyspnea (especially with exertion), edema palpitations, presyncope or syncope, recent change in symptoms
Prior cardiac testing (stress studies, ECG, echo, catheterization)	Dates and results
Medication review	Obtain a careful medication list, including recent/frequency of nitroglycerin use, beta-blockers, antiplatelets, and statins. Specifically ask about medication compliance
Primary cardiologist	Communicate with cardiologist, especially when patient is at high risk for cardiac complications and/or antiplatelet therapy is being held

- If surgery is urgent, discuss case directly with the anesthesia team, and consider engaging a cardiac anesthesiologist in patients with severe coronary disease.

MANAGEMENT OF PATIENTS WITH CARDIAC STENTS

Drug-eluting stents (DES) are commonly used in patients with CAD and can present challenges perioperatively if recently placed. Drug-eluting stents have a modest incidence (1.3 %) of stent thrombosis when antiplatelet therapy is withheld, with serious potential outcomes (50–70 % risk of myocardial infarction and 10–40 % risk of death) [3]. Dual antiplatelet therapy (DAPT) (e.g., clopidogrel and aspirin) is recommended for a full year after DES placement [4], although several recent trials suggest a shorter duration of DAPT (3–6 months) may be acceptable. Sample sizes were too small to generate broad confidence with this approach [5, 6]. In some high-risk cases, dual antiplatelet therapy is extended beyond 12 months. Thus, the usual recommendation is to avoid elective procedures within the first year following stent placement, unless they can be performed without stopping aspirin and clopidogrel.

In general, bare metal stents (BMS) have higher rates of restenosis than DES. However, when DAPT is stopped for any reason within a year of stent placement, there is a substantially higher risk of stent thrombosis in DES. Thus, BMS are often considered in patients for whom nonelective surgery (requiring cessation of DAPT) is anticipated within the year. The current recommendation is to delay elective surgery for at least 4–6 weeks after BMS placement.

If urgent or emergent surgery must be performed within the above windows, strongly consider the risks and benefits of withholding antiplatelet agents and work with the surgeon, patients, and cardiologist to determine appropriate timing to resume these medications.

Placement of stents preoperatively strictly to mitigate perioperative cardiovascular risk is rarely recommended, because the potential risk of complications appears to be greater than the benefit of the revascularization [7]. However, American College of Cardiology/American Heart Association (ACC/AHA) guidelines do recommend consideration for revascularization prior to elective surgery in patients with symptomatic disease, such as unstable angina with significant lesions (especially left main) and patients with unstable cardiac disease [2]. In patients with active symptoms of ischemic heart disease or a positive stress test in whom you are considering perioperative optimization, discuss the case with the patient's cardiologist to weigh potential benefits and risks of revascularization (see Chap. 6 for further discussion).

PERIOPERATIVE MANAGEMENT

MEDICATION MANAGEMENT (ALSO SEE CHAP. 4)

The potential benefits of uninterrupted aspirin (especially in patients with vascular disease) may be higher than the surgical bleeding risk. Our practice is to continue low-dose aspirin (81 mg daily) perioperatively for patients on aspirin for secondary prevention, if the type of surgery allows.

- Studies have shown that cessation of aspirin may result in a transient aspirin withdrawal syndrome, increasing the risk of stroke and MI among patients with cardiovascular disease (especially those patients with indwelling stents) [8].
- The PeriOperative ISchemic Evaluation 2 (POISE-2) study randomized patients to either placebo or aspirin 200 mg daily perioperatively and found no reduction in risk of myocardial infarction or death, but higher risk of major bleeding in the

aspirin group (4.6 % vs. 3.8 %; hazard ratio 1.23; 95 % CI 1.01–1.49; $P = 0.04$) [9].

- The potential risks and benefits of withholding antiplatelet agents perioperatively must be weighed with the patient's primary cardiologist, surgeon, and the patient.
- Stop aspirin 14 days before most neurosurgery, spine, posterior eye, middle ear, and transurethral prostatecomy cases (perioperative bleeding can be a serious challenge).
- Restart aspirin postoperatively as soon as safe from a surgical perspective.
- Stop clopidogrel 5 days (at a minimum) before most surgical interventions.

Continue prescribed beta-blockers and statins perioperatively without interruption, including the morning of surgery. Postoperatively, if the patient is unable to take oral medications, convert beta-blocker to intravenous form.

Resume home antihypertensives postoperatively (with holding parameters); consider holding ACE inhibitors and angiotensin receptor blockers for 24–48 h postoperatively, especially if large fluid shifts and/or hemodynamic instability.

SURVEILLANCE FOR POSTOPERATIVE ISCHEMIA

The PeriOperative ISchemic Evaluation (POISE) investigators conducted a cohort study and found a higher than expected incidence of postoperative MI in high-risk patients (5 %); many of these patients had no symptoms of ischemia [10]. Thus, postoperative monitoring in patients with ischemic heart disease should include:

- Consider telemetry monitoring in patients at highest risk for cardiac complications (including patients with history of ischemia, heart failure, cerebrovascular disease, diabetes, and chronic kidney disease)
- Closely monitor blood pressure and heart rate; if any symptoms or signs of cardiac ischemia, check serial cardiac enzymes and ECG

REFERENCES

1. Lee TH, Marcantonio ER, Mangione CM, et al. Derivation and prospective validation of a simple index for prediction of cardiac risk of major noncardiac surgery. Circulation. 1999;100:1043–9.
2. Fleisher LA, Fleischmann KE, Auerbach AD, et al. 2014 ACC/AHA guideline on perioperative cardiovascular evaluation and management of patients undergoing noncardiac surgery. J Am Coll Cardiol. 2014. doi:10.1016/j.jacc.2014.07.944.
3. Holmes DR, Kereiakes DJ, Garg S, et al. Stent thrombosis. J Am Coll Cardiol. 2010;56(17):1357–65.

4. Vandvik PO, Lincoff AM, Gore JM, et al. Primary and secondary prevention of cardiovascular disease: antithrombotic therapy and prevention of thrombosis, 9th ed: American College of Chest Physicians Evidence-Based Clinical Practice Guidelines. Chest. 2012;141(2 Suppl):e637S.
5. Feres F, Costa RA, Abizaid A, et al. Three vs twelve months of dual antiplatelet therapy after zotarolimus-eluting stents: the OPTIMIZE randomized trial. JAMA. 2013;310(23):2510.
6. Gwon HC, Hahn JY, Park KW, et al. Six-month versus 12-month dual antiplatelet therapy after implantation of drug-eluting stents: the Efficacy of Xience/Promus Versus Cypher to Reduce Late Loss After Stenting (EXCELLENT) randomized, multicenter study. Circulation. 2012;125(3):505–13.
7. McFalls EO, Ward HB, Moritz TE, et al. Coronary-artery revascularization before elective major vascular surgery. N Engl J Med. 2004;351(27):2795–804.
8. Burger W, Chemnitius JM, Kneissl GD, et al. Low dose aspirin for secondary cardiovascular prevention: cardiovascular risks and its perioperative withdrawal versus bleeding risks with its continuation—review and meta-analysis. J Intern Med. 2005;257:399–414.
9. Devereaux PJ, Mrkobrada M, Sessler D. Aspirin in patients undergoing noncardiac surgery. N Engl J Med. 2014;370:1494–503.
10. Devereaux PJ, Xavier D, Pogue J, et al. Characteristics and short-term prognosis of perioperative myocardial infarction in patients undergoing noncardiac surgery: a cohort study. POISE (PeriOperative Ischemic Evaluation) Investigators. Ann Intern Med. 2011;154(8):523.

Chapter 8
Perioperative Beta-Blockers

Paul B. Cornia and Kay M. Johnson

BACKGROUND

Early studies of prophylactic perioperative beta-blockade (i.e., started prior to surgery to reduce adverse cardiovascular outcomes) suggested benefit and led to relatively widespread clinical use. However, a subsequent large randomized controlled trial demonstrated harm and an influential family of trials has now been discredited due to scientific misconduct. This has led to more conservative recommendations.

EARLY STUDIES (PRIOR TO POISE)

In 1996, a randomized trial of 200 patients undergoing major noncardiac surgery with known coronary artery disease (CAD) or multiple risk factors for it found that those who received atenolol beginning immediately before surgery and while hospitalized had reduced mortality at 2 years [1]. However, there were concerns regarding the randomization, lack of intention-to-treat analysis, and the absence of effect in the immediate postoperative period. The Dutch Echocardiographic Cardiac Risk Evaluation Applying Stress Echocardiography (DECREASE) study group performed a small, unblinded study in 1999 in which perioperative treatment with bisoprolol was compared to usual care in patients with a positive dobutamine stress echocardiogram undergoing major vascular surgery [2]. Dramatic reductions in both postoperative cardiac death and nonfatal myocardial infarction were reported. These two trials led to numerous additional studies of perioperative beta-blockade in a variety of surgical populations, most of which showed no benefit. The DECREASE group published several additional influential perioperative beta-blocker trials. However, after extensive investigation, this family of trials has been discredited due to major flaws including the fabrication of data [3–6].

M.B. Jackson et al. (eds.), *The Perioperative Medicine Consult Handbook*, DOI 10.1007/978-3-319-09366-6_8,
© Springer International Publishing Switzerland 2015

POISE TRIAL TO PRESENT

In 2008, the POISE trial results were published. More than 8,000 beta-blocker naïve patients from 190 hospitals and 23 countries with atherosclerotic vascular disease, or multiple risk factors for it, undergoing major noncardiac surgery were randomly assigned to a regimen of high-dose oral and/or intravenous metoprolol started immediately before and continued after surgery [7]. The risk of cardiovascular death, nonfatal MI, or nonfatal cardiac arrest was decreased in the metoprolol succinate-treated group. However, this benefit was offset by an increased risk of stroke and all-cause mortality possibly due to beta-blocker-induced bradycardia and hypotension. A recent meta-analysis including only "secure" trials (i.e., excluding the DECREASE trials), and dominated by the POISE trial, reported similar findings [6]. Although the dose (100 mg of metoprolol succinate) and the timing (initiated 2–4 h before surgery) of beta-blocker used in the POISE trial may have contributed to the adverse outcomes, the available evidence from the remaining available "secure" trials does not allow identification of specific patients who may benefit or beta-blocker regimens that may be beneficial.

Given concerns about the safety of perioperative beta-blockade, a large, propensity-matched, retrospective cohort study using Veterans Health Administration databases was recently conducted [8]. In patients treated with beta-blockers undergoing noncardiac, nonvascular surgery, overall mortality and cardiac morbidity were reduced without increased risk of stroke. Most patients were receiving long-term beta-blocker therapy, but similar outcomes were also observed in those in whom the beta-blocker was initiated within 30 days of surgery; there was insufficient data to assess the outcomes of patients in whom a beta-blocker was started within 7 days of surgery.

PREOPERATIVE EVALUATION

- Determine if the patient is currently taking a beta-blocker.
- We do not recommend starting beta-blockers prior to surgery solely for prophylactic purposes (i.e., to reduce adverse cardiac outcomes) given concerns about adverse perioperative outcomes (increased stroke and mortality).
- The recent ACC/AHA and European Society of Cardiology (ESC) guidelines [9, 10] on perioperative cardiac care list indications in which prophylactic perioperative beta-blocker therapy may be considered (i.e., class IIb; such as myocardial ischemia on a cardiac stress test or ≥3 Revised Cardiac Risk

Index risk factors); however, others have strongly argued against this [11]. Because the current evidence indicates a higher risk for harm with prophylactic perioperative blockade, particularly increased all-cause mortality, it is not our practice to start a beta-blocker in these situations.

- The preoperative medical evaluation is an opportunity to not only improve perioperative outcomes, but also the long-term health of patients. On occasion, a patient may not be on beta-blocker therapy (e.g., stopped it on their own or was never prescribed) despite a class I indication independent of the planned surgery (e.g., stable CAD with history of myocardial infarction or acute coronary syndrome within the past 3 years or for treatment of angina) [12]. In these cases, initiation of a beta-blocker is appropriate for medical optimization and the long-term health benefits, but we believe it should be done at least weeks in advance of surgery with appropriate follow-up prior to the surgery to ensure that bradycardia and/or hypotension do not develop.

PERIOPERATIVE MANAGEMENT

- If the patient is taking a beta-blocker, continue it perioperatively, including the morning of surgery. This is the only class I indication (i.e., recommended) for perioperative beta-blocker therapy [9, 10].
- Abrupt withdrawal of beta-blockade postoperatively may precipitate adverse cardiac events and is associated with increased postoperative mortality [8, 13, 14]. However, specific postoperative clinical circumstances (e.g., bradycardia, hypotension, bleeding) may necessitate that the beta-blocker dosage be modified or that it be temporarily discontinued [10].
- If the patient is unable to take medications by mouth postoperatively, substitute an intravenous formulation (e.g., metoprolol IV every 6 h; dosage may be titrated based on heart and blood pressure response).

REFERENCES

1. Mangano DT, Layug EL, Wallace A, et al. Effect of atenolol on mortality and cardiovascular morbidity after noncardiac surgery. N Engl J Med. 1996; 335:1713–20.
2. Poldermans D, Boersma E, Bax JJ, et al. The effect of bisoprolol on perioperative mortality and myocardial infarction in high-risk patients undergoing vascular surgery. N Engl J Med. 1999;341:1789–94.

3. Erasmus Medical Centre. Investigation into possible violation of scientific integrity. 2011. http://www.erasmusmc.nl/5663/135857/3664573/3397899/report_summary_investigation_integrity. Accessed 13 Jan 2014.

4. Erasmus Medical Centre. Report on the 2012 follow-up investigation of possible breaches of academic integrity. 2012. http://cardiobrief.files.wordpress.com/2012/10/integrity-report-2012-10-english-translation.pdf. Accessed 13 Jan 2014.

5. Chopra V, Eagle KA. Perioperative mischief: the price of academic misconduct. Am J Med. 2012;125:953–5.

6. Bouri S, Shun-Shin MJ, Cole GD, Mayet J, Francis DP. Meta-analysis of secure randomised controlled trials of β-blockade to prevent perioperative death in non-cardiac surgery. Heart. 2013;100:456–64.

7. Devereaux PJ, Yang H, POISE Study Group, et al. Effects of extended-release metoprolol succinate in patients undergoing non-cardiac surgery (POISE trial): a randomised controlled trial. Lancet. 2008;371:1839–47.

8. London MJ, Hur K, Schwartz GG, Henderson WG. Association of perioperative β-blockade with mortality and cardiovascular morbidity following major noncardiac surgery. JAMA. 2013;309:1704–13.

9. Fleisher LA, Fleischmann KE, Auerbach AD, Barnason SA, Beckman JA, Bozkurt B, Davila-Roman VG, Gerhard-Herman MD, Holly TA, Kane GC, Marine JE, Nelson MT, Spencer CC, Thompson A, Ting HH, Uretsky BF, Wijeysundera DN. 2014 ACC/AHA guideline on perioperative cardiovascular evaluation and management of patients undergoing noncardiac surgery. J Am Coll Cardiol. 2014. doi: 10.1016/j.jacc.2014.07.944.

10. Joint Task Force on Non-Cardiac Surgery Cardiovascular Assessment and Management of the European Society of Cardiology (ESC) and the European Society of Anaesthesiology (ESA). 2014 ESC/ESA guidelines on non-cardiac surgery: cardiovascular assessment and management. Eur Heart J. 2014;35(35): 2383–431.

11. Cole GD, Francis DP. Perioperative β blockade: guidelines do not reflect the problems with the evidence from the DECREASE trials. BMJ. 2014;349:g5210. doi:10.1136/bmj.g5210.

12. Fihn SD, Gardin JM, Abrams J, et al. 2012 ACCF/AHA/AATS/PCNA/SCAI/STS guideline for the diagnosis and management of patients with stable ischemic heart disease: a report of the American College of Cardiology Foundation/American Heart Association task force on practice guidelines, and the American College of Physicians, American Association for Thoracic Surgery, Preventive Cardiovascular Nurses Association, Society for Cardiovascular Angiography and Interventions, and Society of Thoracic Surgeons. Circulation. 2012;126:e354.

13. Wallace AW, Au S, Cason BA. Association of the pattern of use of perioperative beta-blockade and postoperative mortality. Anesthesiology. 2010;113:794–805.

14. Kwon S, Thompson R, Florence M, Surgical Care and Outcomes Assessment Program (SCOAP) Collaborative. Beta-blocker continuation after noncardiac surgery: a report from the surgical care and outcomes assessment program. Arch Surg. 2012;147(5):467–73.

Chapter 9
Atrial Fibrillation

Kay M. Johnson and Paul B. Cornia

BACKGROUND

Atrial fibrillation is commonly encountered by the medical consultant, in patients with preexisting atrial fibrillation as well as those with a new onset in the postoperative period. Balancing the risk of stroke versus the risk of bleeding complications is required for the perioperative management of anticoagulation. Strategies for maintaining rate and/or rhythm control must be considered.

PREOPERATIVE EVALUATION

FOR PATIENTS WITH PREEXISTING ATRIAL FIBRILLATION
- Determine whether the atrial fibrillation is paroxysmal versus persistent.
- Review medication list with the patient, noting rate-controlling agents, antiarrhythmics, anticoagulants, or antiplatelet agents.
- Identify any history of rheumatic valvular heart disease, heart failure, hypertension, transient ischemic attack (TIA), or stroke.
- Review prior echocardiogram(s).
- Review previous management of interruptions in anticoagulant therapy, including prior use of bridge heparin therapy (see below).
- Perform a complete cardiovascular examination (heart rate, cardiac murmurs, signs of heart failure) and an electrocardiogram (ECG).
- Estimate the risk for arterial thromboembolism (e.g., using $CHADS_2$ scoring system, see below) [1].

M.B. Jackson et al. (eds.), *The Perioperative Medicine Consult Handbook*, DOI 10.1007/978-3-319-09366-6_9,
© Springer International Publishing Switzerland 2015

- Per American College of Cardiology/American Heart Association (ACC/AHA) guidelines, a supraventricular arrhythmia with a heart rate >100 beats per minute at rest is considered an "active cardiac condition" that should be addressed prior to surgery (see Chap. 6).

PERIOPERATIVE MANAGEMENT

PREOPERATIVE MANAGEMENT
Key issues for the medicine consultant include optimal perioperative rate and rhythm control, and management of anticoagulation, which may include antiplatelet agents, warfarin, or newer oral anticoagulants.

Rhythm and Rate Control
AV nodal blockers are typically continued perioperatively, and a postop plan should be made for continuing these agents, taking into account whether the patient is anticipated to be able to take oral medications (See Table 9.1). For patients receiving less commonly used medications such as sotalol, propafenone, and amiodarone, consider discussing management with the patient's cardiologist.

Management of Antiplatelet Agents
Decisions about antiplatelet agents preoperatively should take into account potential risks and benefits of aspirin cessation; management is increasingly deferred to the individual practices of the surgical team. When it is necessary to discontinue aspirin, aspirin/dipyridamole, or clopidogrel for surgery, they are generally held for 7 days prior to surgery. Consider holding antiplatelet agents longer (up to 14 days) for specific cases, including neuro/spine surgery. When the patient also has significant cardiovascular disease, especially recently implanted coronary stents, consider discussing antiplatelet management with the patient's cardiologist (see Chap. 7).

Warfarin Anticoagulation and Heparin Bridge Therapy
For most surgical procedures, warfarin must be interrupted perioperatively (see below for exceptions), leaving the patient without anticoagulation for several days. A decision must be made about whether "bridging" with heparin is warranted to minimize the duration of the interruption in anticoagulation. A multidisciplinary approach to this decision is recommended, involving the patient, perioperative medicine consultant, surgeon, and anesthesiologist, as well as the

TABLE 9.1 POSTOPERATIVE MANAGEMENT OF PATIENTS WITH PREEXISTING ATRIAL FIBRILLATION

Rate control	If NPO
	Individualize desired rate control target, depending on the patient's baseline rate control goals, the presence of ischemic heart disease, and the patient's post-op blood pressure. In most cases, a heart rate of 70–100 is reasonable
	Metoprolol IV (start 5 mg IV q 6 h and individualize dosing)
	OR
	Diltiazem IV infusion
	Continue digoxin (IV) if receiving digoxin pre-op
	Transition to PO meds when tolerating a diet
	For patients taking a diet
	In most cases, resume patient's usual outpatient rate control regimen. Watch for hypotension since some patients are relatively volume depleted and the blood pressure-lowering effect of some rate control medications may be less well tolerated initially post-op
Anticoagulation	Resume anticoagulation when surgically acceptable (see Chap. 18)
	Bridge with heparin, if indicated, until therapeutic on warfarin
	If anticoagulation is not started immediately due to bleeding risk, venous thromboembolism prophylaxis should still be given, unless there is a contraindication

clinicians managing the patient's anticoagulation in the outpatient setting (e.g., primary care provider, anticoagulation clinic). Develop a plan for perioperative anticoagulation prior to surgery whenever possible. Discuss the plan with the patient, provide written instructions, and clearly document the plan in the medical record. The plan should anticipate postoperative conditions affecting resumption of anticoagulation. Chapter 18 details our approach to bridging anticoagulation, which is based on the 2012 American College of Chest Physicians (ACCP) Guidelines [2].

Note that warfarin need not be stopped for certain low-risk procedures, e.g., dental extractions, dermatologic procedures, and cataract surgery. Ensure that the surgeon is in agreement with this plan and that the pre-op INR is <3.0. Some issues specific to bridging for atrial fibrillation are presented here:

2012 ACCP Practice Guidelines

- These guidelines offer recommendations for perioperative anticoagulation management based on observational data and clinical experience [2].
- The guidelines use the $CHADS_2$ scoring system to estimate stroke risk (see footnote to Table 9.3 in this chapter for details on how the $CHADS_2$ is calculated).
- For patients at low risk of stroke ($CHADS_2$ score = 0–2, assuming no prior stroke/TIA), bridge heparin is not recommended.
- For patients at high risk for perioperative thromboembolism (defined as $CHADS_2$ score = 5–6, stroke/TIA within the past 3 months or associated rheumatic valvular heart disease), bridge heparin is recommended.
- For patients at moderate risk ($CHADS_2$ score = 3–4), the limited data do not allow a specific approach to be recommended for all patients; patient and surgery-specific factors should be assessed on a case-by-case basis. This is a change from prior ACCP guidelines which suggested bridging for $CHADS_2$ score 3–4. As an example of surgery-specific factors to take into account, the current guidelines recommend providers consider not bridging these moderate-risk patients if undergoing high bleeding risk procedures, including major cardiac surgery or carotid endarterectomy.

CHA_2DS_2-VASc Score

- A newer stroke risk prediction tool, the CHA_2DS_2-VASc score, adds female gender, age 65–74, and history of vascular disease to the scoring [3].
- Whether it is more predictive of stroke risk than $CHADS_2$ is being investigated.
- It may be helpful in further defining the risk of stroke in patients with a $CHADS_2$ score 0–1, a group that is already at low-enough risk not to warrant bridging.

Bridging Strategies

- In most cases, warfarin is held for 5 days (five doses) prior to surgery.
- Individualize the number of days that anticoagulation will be held pre-op based on the type of surgery (e.g., neurosurgery, spine surgery, and highly vascular tumors may require a longer period off of anticoagulation), the surgeon's preference, and

the baseline dose of warfarin (patients requiring lower doses tend to have INRs that normalize more slowly).

■ Do not assume that outpatient procedures are low risk for post-procedure surgical bleeding (e.g., angioembolization). Discuss with the surgeon or interventionalist.

■ For details on how to manage bridging and the pros and cons of LMW heparin versus IV unfractionated heparin, see Chap. 18.

Management of Recently Approved Anticoagulants

Dabigatran is an alternative to warfarin for the prevention of stroke in patients with atrial fibrillation. It is an oral direct competitive inhibitor of factor IIa (thrombin) that does not require coagulation monitoring nor bridging with heparin when interrupted [4]. Its clearance is affected by renal function, and though it is not metabolized by the cytochrome P450 (CYP3A4) system, dabigatran still has many drug interactions (including dronedarone, ketoconazole, amiodarone, verapamil, quinidine, and rifampin) [5, 6]. Contraindications include a prosthetic heart valve or hemodynamically significant valve disease, severe renal failure (CrCl <15 mL/min), or advanced liver disease (impaired baseline clotting function) [5]. It is generally not recommended for CrCl less than 30.

Dabigatran should be held 1–4 days prior to surgery, depending on the risk of perioperative bleeding and the patient's renal function. For surgeries with a "standard" risk of bleeding, recommendations are to hold for at least 24 h for CrCl > 50 mL/min and at least 48 h for CrCl 30–50 mL/min. For surgeries with a high risk of bleeding or in which complete hemostasis is required (including abdominal, cardiac, neurosurgery, any major organ surgery, and the use of spinal anesthesia), hold dabigatran for 2–4 days in patients with CrCl > 50 mL/min and 4 days for CrCl 30–50 mL/min [4, 6] (see also Chap. 18).

Unlike warfarin, the anticoagulant effect of dabigatran begins within 2–3 h of the first dose when it is resumed [4]. No antidote to dabigatran is available in the event of bleeding. Its clearance is somewhat hastened by dialysis, but the use of dialysis to help manage a bleeding complication would only be recommended in patients who are already receiving dialysis.

Rivaroxaban and apixaban are oral direct factor Xa inhibitors approved for stroke prevention in nonvalvular atrial fibrillation [7, 8]. Dosing is adjusted for renal function. Like dabigatran, they do not require monitoring or bridging with heparin. There are no reversal agents for these medications and they cannot be dialyzed [5]. Each is held 24 h prior to procedures with standard risk of bleeding or 24–48 h before procedures with high risk of bleeding [6].

POSTOPERATIVE MANAGEMENT

Recommendations for the postoperative management of patients with preexisting atrial fibrillation are summarized in Table 9.1. Review the initial plan for resumption of anticoagulation. Adjustments may be necessary, depending on the surgeon's assessment of the patient's bleeding risk or if unanticipated complications arise. If therapeutic anticoagulation is not restarted immediately postoperatively, patients should still receive venous thromboembolism chemoprophylaxis unless there is an absolute contraindication. Patients should be monitored for embolic complications.

Prevention of Postoperative Atrial Fibrillation

In cardiac surgery, postoperative atrial fibrillation is common. According to the 2014 ACC/AHA/Heart Rhythm Society (HRS) guidelines for the management of atrial fibrillation [9], preoperative administration of amiodarone reduces the incidence of atrial fibrillation in patients undergoing cardiac surgery and is reasonable for prophylactic therapy in patients at high risk for atrial fibrillation. Prophylactic sotalol or colchicine may also be considered for patients undergoing cardiac surgery, and statins may be beneficial in patients undergoing coronary revascularization [9]. Use of medications for atrial fibrillation prevention is usually deferred to the cardiac surgeon.

In noncardiac surgery, three small randomized trials have studied prophylactic amiodarone use in thoracic surgery patients (lung resection surgery, lung cancer surgery, and esophagectomy). All three studies showed a reduction in post-op atrial fibrillation [10]. Current practice guidelines do not offer specific recommendations on the use of amiodarone for this indication.

Management of New-Onset Postoperative Atrial Fibrillation

- Identify precipitating causes (e.g., heart failure, electrolyte imbalance, infection, infarction, alcohol withdrawal, thyroid abnormalities, anemia, hypovolemia, lung disease, valvular heart disease, pulmonary embolism, volume overload/reabsorbed third-spaced fluids, etc.).
- Assess how well the patient is tolerating the arrhythmia: symptoms, hypotension, and evidence of heart failure or ischemia.
- Obtain an echocardiogram to assess left ventricular EF and look for valvular heart disease.
- Rate control for atrial fibrillation with rapid ventricular response: Generally start with IV agents if rate control is needed urgently. Use caution when considering beta-blockers and

TABLE 9.2 RATE CONTROL STRATEGIES FOR NEW-ONSET POST-OP ATRIAL FIBRILLATION WITH RAPID VENTRICULAR RESPONSE

Metoprolol	5 mg IV × 1. May repeat ×2 if additional rate control needed and BP remains stable
Diltiazem	Bolus 10–20 mg IV, then start IV infusion at 10–20 mg/h, titrate to HR 80–100
Digoxin	Acts more slowly. 0.5 mg IV × 1, then 0.25 mg IV Q6H ×2 Give daily and titrate to effect; typical dose is 0.125 mg IV or PO daily Reduce dose if renal dysfunction. Use caution in elderly patients
Amiodarone	150 mg IV bolus, then load with 1 mg/min IV × 6 h, then 0.5 mg/min × 18 h Indicated for refractory atrial fibrillation or atrial fibrillation with heart failure Check baseline TSH, PFTs
Esmolol	50–300 mcg/kg/min IV. Can bolus 500 mcg/kg IV initially Watch for hypotension
PO medications	Multiple options: metoprolol, atenolol, or diltiazem Digoxin or amiodarone, if indicated
Cardioversion	Immediate cardioversion is indicated if hemodynamically unstable. Must address anticoagulation

calcium channel blockers in patients with heart failure or hypotension (see Table 9.2).

Post-op atrial fibrillation often resolves spontaneously, or there may be brief, self-limited episodes of atrial fibrillation that resolve once the postoperative stress resolves; anticoagulation is generally not necessary for these patients. When atrial fibrillation persists or continues to recur, antithrombotic therapy (i.e., antiplatelet or anticoagulant) should be considered for patients at increased risk of stroke:

- The CHADS$_2$ score (Table 9.3) is commonly used as a risk stratification tools used in practice [1, 11].
- This decision should be made on an individual basis, taking into consideration the patient's risk factors and personal goals as much as possible. Consultation with the patient's primary care provider may be helpful.
- For high-risk patients with atrial fibrillation deemed unsuitable for anticoagulation, dual antiplatelet therapy with clopidogrel

TABLE 9.3 CHADS$_2$ RISK STRATIFICATION FOR ATRIAL FIBRILLATION

Score	Annual stroke risk	Recommended anticoagulation
0	1.9	ASA
1	2.8	ASA or warfarin
2	4.0	Warfarin
3	5.9	Warfarin
4+	>7 %	Warfarin

Scoring: 1 point for CHF, HTN, Age > 75, DM; 2 points for a history of TIA/CVA. However, if the CHADS$_2$ score is 2 because of a history of TIA/CVA, the annual stroke risk is likely *greater* than 4 %

Adapted with permission from [11]

and aspirin can be considered; this offers more protection against stroke than aspirin alone but with an increased risk of major bleeding [11].

When rhythm control is considered, it is advisable to obtain cardiology consultation to advise on issues around pharmacologic and electrical cardioversion and potential need for transesophageal echocardiogram to decrease the risk of cardioembolic stroke. Key points for the medicine consultant include:

- Amiodarone is often used but has a very long half-life and may cause significant long-term side effects.
- Dronedarone is a newer agent with potentially less pulmonary and thyroid side effects compared with amiodarone. However, it is only available orally and should be avoided in patients with heart failure and may increase cardiovascular events in high-risk patients with permanent atrial fibrillation; it is not advised in new-onset post-op atrial fibrillation pending resolution of these safety concerns.
- Other antiarrhythmic agents (such as dofetilide, flecainide, propafenone, and sotalol) and cardioversion may be considered in consultation with a cardiologist.

REFERENCES

1. Gage BF, Waterman AD, Shannon W, Boechler M, Rich MW, Radford MJ. Validation of clinical classification schemes for predicting stroke: results from the National Registry of Atrial Fibrillation. JAMA. 2001;285(22):2864.
2. Douketis JD, Spyropoulos AC, Spencer FA, et al. Perioperative management of antithrombotic therapy: antithrombotic therapy and prevention of thrombosis, 9th edition: American College of Chest Physicians Evidence-Based Clinical Practice Guidelines. Chest. 2012;141 (2 Suppl):e326s–50s.

3. Lip GY, Nieuwlaat R, Pisters R, Lane DA, Crijns HJ. Refining clinical risk stratification for predicting stroke and thromboembolism in atrial fibrillation using a novel risk factor-based approach: the euro heart survey on atrial fibrillation. Chest. 2010;137(2):263–72.
4. van Ryn J, Stangier J, Haertter S, et al. Dabigatran etexilate—a novel, reversible, oral direct thrombin inhibitor: interpretation of coagulation assays and reversal of anticoagulant activity. Thromb Haemost. 2010;103:1116–27.
5. Furie KL, Goldstein LB, Albers GW, et al. Oral antithrombotic agents for the prevention of stroke in nonvalvular atrial fibrillation: a science advisory for healthcare professionals from the American Heart Association/American Stroke Association. Stroke. 2012;43:3442–53.
6. University of Washington Medical Center Anticoagulation Clinic website: http://depts.washington.edu/anticoag/home. Accessed 24 Feb 2014.
7. Patel MR, Mahaffey KW, Garg J, et al. Rivaroxaban versus warfarin in nonvalvular atrial fibrillation. N Engl J Med. 2011;365:883–91.
8. Granger CB, Alexander JH, McMurray JJV. Apixaban versus warfarin in patients with atrial fibrillation. N Engl J Med. 2011;365:981–92.
9. January CT, Wann LS, Alpert JS, et al. 2014 AHA/ACC/HRS guideline for the management of patients with atrial fibrillation. J Am Coll Cardiol. 2014. doi:10.1016/j.jacc.2014.03.022.
10. Fleisher LA, Fleischmann KE, Auerbach AD, et al. 2014 ACC/AHA guideline on perioperative cardiovascular evaluation and management of patients undergoing noncardiac surgery. J Am Coll Cardiol. 2014. doi:10.1016/j.jacc.2014.07.944.
11. Goldstein LB, Adams R, Alberts MJ, et al. Primary prevention of ischemic stroke: a guideline from the American Heart Association/American Stroke Association Stroke Council. Circulation. 2006;113:e873–923.

Chapter 10
Hypertension

Nason P. Hamlin and Gail A. Van Norman

BACKGROUND

Hypertension is not a significant risk factor for major adverse cardiac events, but it is a significant risk factor for intraoperative blood pressure lability and the incidence of perioperative myocardial ischemia [1, 2]. These are major reasons for perioperative medical consultation concerning uncontrolled hypertension.

PREOPERATIVE EVALUATION

- Assess level of blood pressure control
- Avoid elective surgery in patients with hypertensive urgency or emergency
- Assess for complications of long-standing hypertension (stroke, hypertensive cardiomyopathy, and nephropathy)
- Consider delaying elective surgery in patients with poorly controlled HTN, e.g., BP > 180/110
- Advise preoperative medication management—see Table 10.1

PERIOPERATIVE MANAGEMENT

OPTIMIZING BLOOD PRESSURE RISK PREOPERATIVELY

The traditional cutoff of deferring surgery if blood pressure is greater than 180/110 is not well supported by contemporary data [1, 2], but many anesthesiologists would be reluctant to take a patient into the operating room for elective surgery with a systolic BP > 180 or a

M.B. Jackson et al. (eds.), *The Perioperative Medicine Consult Handbook*, DOI 10.1007/978-3-319-09366-6_10,
© Springer International Publishing Switzerland 2015

TABLE 10.1 PREOPERATIVE MANAGEMENT OF ANTIHYPERTENSIVE MEDICATIONS

Beta-blockers	Continue, and take on the morning of surgery
ACE inhibitors	Hold on the morning of surgery unless patient has poorly controlled HTN at baseline, e.g., SBP > 180 or DBP > 110
ARBs	Hold on the morning of surgery unless patient has poorly controlled HTN at baseline as above with ACE inhibitors
Diuretics	Hold on the morning of surgery
Calcium channel blockers	Consider holding on the morning of surgery if BP is tightly controlled
Clonidine	Continue, and take on the morning of surgery Transition to clonidine transdermal preoperatively if expected to be NPO postoperatively

diastolic BP > 110. Some studies show that this may be associated with a modest increase in the risk of perioperative stroke. There are no good data that say, however, that deferring surgery for definitive blood pressure control is superior to acute blood pressure control in the preoperative holding area. Blood pressure risk is a continuum and must be balanced by many factors, including the urgency of surgery. Medications can be given in the preop holding area to ameliorate the high pressure without having to cancel surgery. It is best to work with the anesthesiologist.

There are some surgical procedures (such as facial plastic surgery and intraocular surgery) that should not be done without better control of hypertension because of the risks of increased intraoperative bleeding. On the other hand, acutely lowering blood pressure in patients with certain types of problems, such as patients with high intracranial pressure, is more dangerous than leaving things alone, even if significant hypertension is present. Again, work with your anesthesiology colleagues to optimize blood pressure in the context of the patient's comorbidities and the planned surgery.

It is important to understand what happens in the intraoperative phase controlled by the anesthesia team. Intraop SBP can average 50 mmHg below ambulatory levels; tight control preop may lead to profound hypotension intraop requiring pressors and extra fluids. Preoperative medication management strategies may minimize the risk of intraoperative hypotension:

- It is reasonable to hold angiotensin-converting enzyme (ACE) inhibitors and angiotensin receptor blockers (ARBs) on the morning of surgery unless the systolic BP is >180 or the

TABLE 10.2 IV AND TRANSDERMAL OPTIONS FOR TREATING HYPERTENSION

Metoprolol	5 mg IV q 4–6 h. Titrate to desired BP and HR
Labetalol	20–80 mg IV q 5–10 min (up to 300 mg)
Nitroglycerin	IV drip 5 mcg/min, titrate to desired BP
	1–2″ ointment q 6 h (works more slowly than drip)
Hydralazine	20 mg IV. Repeat after 20 min if needed. If still no effect, try another agent. Caution in patients with CAD
Esmolol	500 mcg/kg for the first minute, then 50–300 mcg/kg/min. Use only if minute-to-minute titration is needed Longer-acting drugs are usually preferred
Nicardipine	More commonly used in neurosurgical patients

diastolic BP is >110. This practice remains controversial—the evidence is conflicting and based on small studies or retrospective cohorts.

- Our practice is to hold diuretics on the morning of surgery. While the risk of taking the diuretic is theoretical, there is also no clear advantage in patients who are taking a diuretic for hypertension to take it on the morning of surgery. One small study showed no difference in outcomes [3].

POSTOPERATIVE MANAGEMENT OF ANTIHYPERTENSIVES

Low blood pressures are common postop due to blood loss, sedation, pain medications, and bed rest. Conversely, mild to moderate BP elevations, especially in patients not previously hypertensive, usually do not require treatment. There are several important considerations in choosing blood pressure medications postoperatively.

- *NPO status*: Consider the patient's preoperative home medications, and whether the patient can take PO medications or must remain strictly NPO. Postoperative patients are often NPO for prolonged periods of time. Often a patient's bowel function has returned enough to absorb critical medications, even if the patient is not yet on a full diet—discussion with the surgery team is essential.
- *IV and transdermal treatment*: Nitroglycerin is favored over hydralazine in patients with coronary artery disease. IV metoprolol and labetalol are useful for blood pressure control in patients who are NPO—however, they must be given with caution in patients with severe asthma and generally avoided in decompensated heart failure. Table 10.2 shows IV/transdermal options for treating hypertension.

TABLE 10.3 MANAGEMENT OF ANTIHYPERTENSIVE MEDICATIONS POSTOP

Beta-blockers	Continue, but hold or reduce if symptomatic hypotension or bradycardia. Common hold parameters are for SBP < 100 or HR < 60, but need to individualize these for each patient
ACE inhibitors and ARBs	If given only for HTN, often do not restart if SBP remains below 120 postop
Diuretics	Consider holding for the first few days postop after major surgery—patients are at risk of hypovolemia and hyponatremia
Clonidine	Continue either PO or transdermal to avoid rebound HTN
Calcium channel blockers	Continue, but hold or reduce if hypotension or bradycardia

- *Postop hypertension*: Assess for underlying cause—pain, alcohol withdrawal, beta-blocker or clonidine withdrawal, essential hypertension, or measurement error. Tremor and postop shivering can cause falsely high blood pressure readings with electronic BP cuffs; it is best to confirm very high readings with a manual cuff and stethoscope in both arms.
- *Resume home blood pressure medications with caution* (see Table 10.3 for recommendations regarding resumption of blood pressure medications postop).

REFERENCES

1. Spahn DR, Priebe HJ. Preoperative hypertension: remain wary? "Yes" cancel surgery? "No". Br J Anaesth. 2004;92(4):461–4.
2. Howell SJ, Sear JW, Foex P. Hypertension, hypertensive heart disease and perioperative risk. Br J Anaesth. 2004;92(4):570–83.
3. Khan NA, Campbell NR, Frost SD, et al. Risk of intraoperative hypotension with loop diuretics: a randomized controlled trial. Am J Med. 2010;123:1059e1–8.

Chapter 11
Valvular Heart Disease

Divya Gollapudi

BACKGROUND

Severe valvular disease is identified as a cardiac risk factor in the American College of Cardiology/American Heart Association (ACC/AHA) perioperative guidelines, requiring evaluation and management prior to noncardiac surgery [1, 2]. Attention to the type and severity of valvular heart disease during the preoperative visit can help guide perioperative risk assessment and management. Severe aortic stenosis and mitral stenosis are considered to pose the greatest perioperative risk [1, 2]. Distinguishing pathologic from functional murmurs and assessing a patient's functional status by careful history and exam are the first essential steps. An echocardiogram should be obtained preoperatively if symptoms or exam are concerning for severe valvular disease.

Perioperative considerations in patients with other structural heart conditions, such as congenital cyanotic heart disease, are beyond the scope of this book—the patient's cardiologist should generally be involved in the care of these patients.

AORTIC STENOSIS

PREOPERATIVE EVALUATION

Aortic stenosis (AS) is a common valvular abnormality in elderly adults [3, 4]. Symptoms include angina, exertional syncope, dyspnea, and decreased exercise tolerance; coronary artery disease is a common comorbidity. The murmur of AS is systolic, located at the right second intercostal space, and can radiate to the right carotid or

M.B. Jackson et al. (eds.), *The Perioperative Medicine
Consult Handbook*, DOI 10.1007/978-3-319-09366-6_11,
© Springer International Publishing Switzerland 2015

TABLE 11.1 ECHOCARDIOGRAPHIC SEVERITY FOR AORTIC STENOSIS

Stage	Aortic jet velocity (m/s)	Mean gradient (mmHg)	Valve area (cm²)
Mild	<3.0	<25	>1.5
Moderate	3.0–4.0	25–40	1.0–1.5
Severe	>4.0	>40	<1.0

clavicular area. Physical examination findings suggestive of severe AS that might warrant preoperative echocardiogram include [5]:

- Late peaking murmur (positive likelihood ratio: +LR 4.4)
- Sustained apical pulse (+LR 4.1)
- Delayed carotid artery upstroke (+LR 3.3)
- Brachioradial delay (+LR 2.5)

Table 11.1 shows severity classification by echocardiogram. In AS, the average decrease in valve area is approximately 0.1 cm² per year, but progression is unpredictable and can occur rapidly [6]. In addition to new or worsening symptoms in a patient known to have AS, it is reasonable to obtain an echocardiogram within:

- 3 months of surgery for asymptomatic with known severe disease
- 6–12 months for moderate disease
- 2 years for mild disease
- 2–3 years for aortic sclerosis

Perioperative Risk Stratification

- Significant AS is associated with increased perioperative mortality; early studies demonstrated a mortality rate of 13% in patients with severe AS undergoing non-cardiac surgery [1, 2].
- Patients with severe aortic stenosis may have impaired platelet function and decreased levels of von Willebrand factor, which can be associated with clinically significant bleeding (usually epistaxis or ecchymoses) [6].
- Aortic sclerosis without stenosis is not considered an independent perioperative risk factor.

PERIOPERATIVE MANAGEMENT
Preoperative Considerations

- Evaluation for valve replacement is recommended in symptomatic patients prior to noncardiac surgery [6].
- Consider cardiology consultation in asymptomatic patients with severe AS.
- Balloon valvotomy is not recommended as a temporizing measure in patients with severe AS undergoing noncardiac surgery [6].

Postoperative Considerations

- For asymptomatic patients with moderate to severe disease: Close postoperative hemodynamic monitoring (up to 48 h), maintenance of intravascular volume, avoidance of tachycardia, and maintenance of sinus rhythm [6, 7].
- In the event of major bleeding or volume loss, maintenance of excellent IV access and rapid resuscitation are vital.
- Avoid the use of nitrates in patients with severe or critical aortic stenosis, as nitrates reduce filling pressures and may precipitate cardiac arrest.
- Patients with subaortic stenosis (i.e., idiopathic hypertrophic subaortic stenosis) should be managed similarly to patients with aortic stenosis.

MITRAL STENOSIS

PREOPERATIVE EVALUATION

Patients with mitral stenosis are at increased risk for perioperative tachyarrhythmias and heart failure; thus, it is important to identify these patients preoperatively [1]. The most common cause of mitral stenosis is rheumatic fever, and common symptoms are dyspnea, decreased exercise tolerance, fatigue, and palpitations. Mitral stenosis causes a low-pitched, blowing diastolic murmur, which is best heard with the bell of the stethoscope [5]. Findings of increasingly severe mitral stenosis include:

- Faint or inaudible murmur [5]
- Diminished S1

PERIOPERATIVE MANAGEMENT

- Preoperative surgical correction of asymptomatic mitral valve disease is generally not indicated prior to noncardiac surgery [1, 6].
- Percutaneous or surgical repair should be considered in patients with severe mitral stenosis who have symptoms and/or severe pulmonary hypertension [1, 6].
- Perioperative heart rate control should be considered, as tachycardia can reduce diastolic filling and lead to pulmonary congestion; discussion with a cardiologist is warranted [1, 6].
- Mitral stenosis leads to a fixed stroke volume, making it important to avoid hypotension and maintain normal systemic vascular resistance [1, 6, 7].
- Perioperative management of atrial fibrillation is discussed in Chap. 9.

AORTIC REGURGITATION

PREOPERATIVE EVALUATION

Limited data suggest that patients with moderate to severe aortic regurgitation (AR) have increased risk of perioperative cardiac and pulmonary morbidity and mortality, as compared to patients without significant AR [8]. Symptoms of chronic AR include palpitations, dyspnea, and chest pain. There are several physical exam findings associated with AR, the most important being the presence of an early, blowing, high-frequency diastolic murmur [5, 9]. Physical exam findings suggestive of moderate to severe AR include [5]:

- Diastolic blood pressure ≤ 50 mmHg (+LR 19.3)
- Pulse pressure ≥ 80 mmHg (+LR 10.9)
- Murmur grade 3 or louder (+LR 8.2)
- S3 gallop (+LR 5.9)

PERIOPERATIVE MANAGEMENT

- Symptomatic patients or asymptomatic patients with significantly reduced left ventricular (LV) function with AR should be considered for valve replacement [6].
- Perioperative management should include attention to volume control and afterload reduction [1].
- Bradycardia should be avoided, as low heart rates can acutely worsen regurgitation by increasing diastolic time [7].

MITRAL REGURGITATION

PREOPERATIVE EVALUATION

Mitral regurgitation (MR) is considered the most common valvular disorder [3]. The most common etiologies are papillary muscle dysfunction from ischemic heart disease and mitral valve prolapse. Recent observational and retrospective studies have reported that patients with severe MR are at greatest risk for perioperative heart failure (20 %) and atrial fibrillation (14 %) [10, 11]—these risks are increased in patients with ischemic MR and decreased LV function [10, 11]. The murmur of MR is holosystolic, high-pitched, and is heard best at the apex. The characteristics of moderate to severe MR include [5]:

- Murmur grade 3 or louder (+LR 4.4)
- S3 (89 % of patients with severe MR)

Echocardiogram Findings
- LV ejection fraction measured on echocardiogram may be overestimated in the setting of severe MR [1, 6].
- Ventricular dysfunction may be present with a normal or only mildly reduced ejection fraction on echocardiogram.

PERIOPERATIVE MANAGEMENT
- Patient with symptomatic MR or asymptomatic MR with significantly decreased LV ejection fraction should be considered for valve repair or replacement [6].
- In patients with severe MR undergoing high-risk procedures, diuretic therapy and afterload reduction should be optimized pre- and postoperatively [1, 7].
- Careful fluid management in patients with even mildly decreased LV function is recommended.
- Bradycardia increases diastolic time and can increase regurgitation, thus should be minimized; however, note that in patients with significant coronary artery disease and ischemic MR, higher heart rates may precipitate demand ischemia [7].
- Antibiotic prophylaxis against infective endocarditis is not recommended for patients with mitral valve prolapse or MR [12, 13].

PROSTHETIC HEART VALVES

PERIOPERATIVE CONSIDERATIONS
Function of the Prosthetic Valve
- Echocardiography is indicated if there is a new murmur, new symptoms, or change in clinical status (including evidence of new or worsening heart failure, hemolytic anemia, systemic embolism) [6, 14].

Management of Anticoagulation
- Anticoagulation in patients with mechanical or bioprosthetic valves requires careful perioperative planning and coordination with the surgical team.
- See Chap. 18 for further discussion of anticoagulation.

Endocarditis Prophylaxis
- The ACC/AHA guidelines recommend endocarditis prophylaxis for patients with certain high-risk cardiac conditions, as shown in Table 11.2 [12].

TABLE 11.2 HIGH-RISK CONDITIONS FOR INFECTIVE ENDOCARDITIS

Prosthetic heart valves or prosthetic material used for cardiac valve repair

History of previous infective endocarditis

Congenital heart disease (CHD) in the following categories
- Unrepaired cyanotic CHD, including palliative shunts and conduits
- Completely repaired congenital heart defect repaired with prosthetic material or device, whether placed by surgery or by catheter intervention, during the first 6 months after the procedure
- Repaired CHD with residual defects at or near the site of a prosthetic patch or device (thus preventing endothelialization)

Cardiac transplantation recipients with valve regurgitation due to structurally abnormal valve

Adapted with permission from [12]

TABLE 11.3 PROCEDURAL INDICATIONS FOR ENDOCARDITIS PROPHYLAXIS

In high-risk patients, endocarditis prophylaxis is recommended for patients undergoing
- All dental procedures involving manipulation of gingival tissue or the periapical region of the teeth or perforation of the oral mucosa
- Respiratory tract procedures involving incision or biopsy of the respiratory mucosa
- Respiratory tract procedures to treat an established infection (e.g., abscess or empyema)
- Procedures involving infected skin, skin structures, or musculoskeletal tissue

Prophylaxis is no longer routinely recommended for
- Routine anesthetic injection through noninfected tissue
- Placement or adjustment of removable prosthodontic or orthodontic appliances or brackets
- Dental radiographs
- Shedding of deciduous teeth
- Bleeding from trauma to the lips or oral mucosa
- Bronchoscopy without mucosal incision
- GI or GU procedures (e.g., EGD/colonoscopy/cystoscopy) (see text for exceptions)

Based on ACC/AHA 2008 guideline update on valvular heart disease: focused update on infective endocarditis [12]

TABLE II.4 ANTIBIOTIC REGIMENS FOR ENDOCARDITIS PROPHYLAXIS IN HIGH-RISK PATIENTS UNDERGOING PROCEDURE-SPECIFIC INDICATIONS

	Antibiotic regimen	Antibiotic regimen if penicillin or ampicillin allergic
Oral	Amoxicillin 2 g	Cephalexin 2 g or Clindamycin 600 mg or Azithromycin 500 mg or Clarithromycin 500 mg
Unable to take oral medication	Ampicillin 2 g IM/IV or Cefazolin 1 g IM/IV or Ceftriaxone 1 g IM/IV	Cefazolin 1 g IM/IV or Ceftriaxone 1 g IM/IV or Clindamycin 600 mg IM/IV

All doses are 30–60 min prior to procedure
Adapted with permission from [12]

- In high-risk patients, endocarditis prophylaxis is recommended for the procedures shown in Table 11.3 [12].
- Prophylaxis should be considered in high-risk patients undergoing gastrointestinal (GI) or genitourinary (GU) procedures, if there is an ongoing infection of GI or GU tract [12].
- Consider antibiotic therapy to eradicate enterococci in patients with an active enterococcal urinary tract infection or colonization before undergoing a GU procedure [12].
- Antibiotic regimens for high-risk patients are listed in Table 11.4 [12].

REFERENCES

1. Fleisher LA, Fleischmann KE, Auerbach AD, et al. 2014 ACC/AHA guideline on perioperative cardiovascular evaluation and management of patients undergoing noncardiac surgery. J Am Coll Cardiol 2014. doi: 10.1016/j.jacc.2014.07.944.
2. Goldman L, Caldera DL, Nussbaum SR, et al. Multifactorial index of cardiac risk in noncardiac surgical procedures. N Engl J Med. 1977;297:845–50.
3. Nkomo VT, Gardin JM, Skelton TN, et al. Burden of valvular heart diseases: a population-based study. Lancet. 2006;368(9540):1005–11.
4. Wright D. Aortic stenosis and surgery. J Hosp Med. 2012;7(8):655–6.
5. McGee S. Evidence-based physical diagnosis. 3rd ed. Philadelphia, PA: Elsevier Saunders; 2012. 736 p.
6. Bonow RO, Carabello BA, Chatterjee K, et al. 2008 Focused update incorporated into the ACC/AHA 2006 guidelines for the management of patients with valvular heart disease: a report of the American College of Cardiology/American Heart Association task force on practice guidelines (Writing Committee to Develop Guidelines for the Management of Patients with Valvular Heart Disease). Circulation. 2008;118:e523–661.
7. Frogel J, Galusca D. Anesthetic considerations for patients with advanced valvular heart disease undergoing noncardiac surgery. Anesthesiol Clin. 2010;28(1):67–85.
8. Lai HC, Lai HC, Lee WL, et al. Impact of chronic advanced aortic regurgitation on the perioperative outcome of noncardiac surgery. Acta Anaesthesiol Scand. 2010;54(5):580–8.

9. Choudhry NK, Etchells EE. The rational clinical examination. Does this patient have aortic regurgitation? JAMA. 1999;281(23):2231–8.

10. Bajaj NS, Agarwal S, Rajamanickam A, et al. Impact of severe mitral regurgitation on postoperative outcomes after noncardiac surgery. Am J Med. 2013;126(6):529–35.

11. Lai HC, Lai HC, Lee WL, et al. Mitral regurgitation complicates postoperative outcome of noncardiac surgery. Am Heart J. 2007;153(4):712–7.

12. Nishimura RA, Carabello BA, Faxon DP, et al. ACC/AHA 2008 guideline update on valvular heart disease: focused update on infective endocarditis. Circulation. 2008;118:887–96.

13. Wilson W, Taubert KA, Gewitz M, et al. Prevention of infective endocarditis: guidelines from the American Heart Association. Circulation. 2007;115:1736–54.

14. Pibarot P, Dumesnil JG. Prosthetic heart valves: selection of the optimal prosthesis and long-term management. Circulation. 2009;119:1034–48.

Chapter 12
Implantable Cardiac Electronic Devices

G. Alec Rooke

BACKGROUND

OVERVIEW OF DEVICE-RELATED COMPLICATIONS

Patients with pacemakers or internal cardioverter-defibrillators (ICDs) are at risk for device malfunction on exposure to electromagnetic interference (EMI) from monopolar cautery, magnetic resonance imaging (MRI), or radiofrequency ablation and therapeutic radiation [1]. The most common and potentially life-threatening adverse effects of EMI are:

- Inhibition of cardiac pacing leading to severe bradycardia or asystole
- Inadvertent shocks if an ICD interprets the EMI as a heart rate higher than the therapy trigger rate

However, EMI may also lead to tachycardia from:

- Noise reversion (when EMI makes the rhythm uninterpretable to the device, the device may automatically switch to asynchronous pacing and thereby create a rhythm that competes with the intrinsic rhythm).
- Activation of the rate-response feature by EMI may cause the pacing rate to increase, which typically results in a paced tachycardia (see below).
- EMI sensed as intrinsic atrial beats that lead to ventricular paced beats.

In addition, if the EMI becomes intense, such as if the cautery occurs within 8 cm of the device, the device may:

- Transiently turn off and when it reboots, revert to default settings instead of the original programmed settings.
- Burn the myocardium at the pacer lead tip if there is a break in the lead insulation.

M.B. Jackson et al. (eds.), *The Perioperative Medicine Consult Handbook*, DOI 10.1007/978-3-319-09366-6_12, © Springer International Publishing Switzerland 2015

TABLE 12.1 PACEMAKER FUNCTION CODES

First letter	Second letter	Third letter
Chamber(s) paced	Chamber(s) sensed	Response to sensing
A = atrium	A = atrium	I = inhibited
V = ventricle	V = ventricle	T = trigger
D = dual (both chambers)	D = dual (both chambers)	D = dual (inhibit or trigger depending on the situation)
	O = no sensing	O = nothing

- If cautery is applied to the device, it may fry the electronics and render the device nonfunctional.

BASIC PACEMAKER AND ICD FUNCTION

Pacemaker function is often summarized with a three- or four-letter code, with the letters designating the chambers that are paced, the chamber(s) where sensing is performed, and the device's response to a sensed beat [2–4] (see Table 12.1). A fourth letter, "R," is often added if a rate-adaptive or rate-responsive mechanism is operational. When the activity sensor within the device determines that the patient is active, the backup (demand) pacing rate increases. Sensor options include the following [5]:

- A piezoelectric crystal that detects either muscle pressure on the device or body movement: In the operating room (OR), shaking the patient can cause increases in heart rate.
- Bioimpedance measurement within the chest to estimate minute ventilation: To make this measurement, the device emits a small current between the generator and the lead. This permits an impedance measurement that reflects tidal volume, and its frequency provides the respiratory rate. The respiratory rate module of most OR/ICU monitors has similar technology and can fool the pacer/implantable cardioverter-defibrillator (ICD) into thinking the patient is physically active. This results in an inappropriate paced tachycardia.
- Bioimpedance measurement within the myocardium (an index of sympathetic nervous system activity): This measurement is made at the tip of the lead. No known interactions in the OR.

MOST COMMON PACING MODES

- *VVI*: Senses and paces the ventricle (demand pacing).
- *DDD*: Both atrium and ventricle are sensed and paced individually.
- *VVIR and DDDR*: Same as VVI or DDD, but with rate-adaptive mechanism.

IMPLANTABLE CARDIOVERTER-DEFIBRILLATORS [2, 3]

- Respond to tachyarrhythmias (typically ventricular tachycardia and fibrillation) based on detection of defined, high ventricular rates.
- Therapies include rapid pacing, low-energy synchronized shocks, or high-energy unsynchronized shocks.
- All ICDs have pacing capability. The pacemaker component of an ICD is the same as a regular pacemaker, and the four-letter code still applies. In an ICD, the pacemaker settings vary from very basic (patient with no need for a pacemaker) to as complex as any patient with pacemaker requirement.

CARDIAC RESYNCHRONIZATION THERAPY

- These devices pace both the right and left ventricles in order to produce a more coordinated left ventricular contraction [2, 3].
- If defibrillation capability is present, it is referred to as CRT-D.
- The four-letter pacing mode nomenclature can still be used to describe the pacemaker capability of the cardiac resynchronization therapy (CRT) or CRT-D device.

PREOPERATIVE EVALUATION

Most experts recommend that a plan for device management for surgery be made by a qualified individual with the recommendation based on knowledge of the proposed surgery and the information gleaned from a recent interrogation of the device [1, 6, 7]. The typical recommendations will be one of the following:

1. Nothing required (e.g., surgery on the leg where EMI detection by the device is virtually unheard of).
2. Place a magnet (fine for an ICD when the cautery is below the umbilicus).
3. A prescription for what programming changes are needed for surgery. If a prescription is needed, then arrangements must be made for a qualified individual to perform the programming.

The decision to proceed with surgery without formal device evaluation should be made cautiously. Clearly the urgency of the surgery is a factor, but the risk of adverse events increases whenever monopolar cautery will be applied within 8 cm of the device, the leads use monopolar sensing (almost all devices use bipolar sensing, but it is almost impossible to know without interrogation), the patient is pacemaker dependent, the ICD is programmed so that it will not respond to a

TABLE 12.2 PACEMAKER COMPANY CONTACT INFORMATION

Company and phone number	Good battery pacemaker magnet rate
Biotronik: (800) 547-0394	90
Ela Sorin: (303) 467-6101	96
Guidant/Boston Scientific: (800) 227-3422	90
Medtronic: (800) 723-4636	85
St. Jude: (800) 933-9956	98.6 or 100

magnet (rare, but potentially disastrous) [8], the device battery is at its end of life, or if the grounding pad is improperly placed.

In the absence of qualified practitioner involvement, there is still a great deal that can be learned without formal device interrogation. Indeed, such analysis can aid in the determination of the need for qualified practitioner involvement [9].

Step 1: Device identification: Pacer or ICD?

- Patients may not know the distinction, but most carry a card with the device and lead(s) model numbers, implant dates, and implanting cardiologist. Also determine when the device was last interrogated. In general, ICDs should have been checked within three months of surgery and pacemakers within six months.

- A chest X-ray provides clear information as to the device and potential pacing capabilities. If all the leads are thin, then the device must be a pacemaker. If some leads have fat, densely radiopaque sections (usually in the superior vena cava and right ventricle), then the device is an ICD.

- Careful scrutiny of the device on the chest X-ray also typically reveals a symbol and letter/number code identifying the manufacturer and model. One can call the manufacturer (see Table 12.2) or check the Web site to obtain information about the device capability including the device's response to a magnet, but the company will not have any patient-specific information.

Step 2: Determine pacer dependency

- Obtain a long rhythm strip or observe on a monitor. This will help to determine the underlying rhythm and if the patient is pacemaker dependent. Make sure that the monitor is set to display pacing spikes. Most modern monitors found in ORs, ERs, and ICUs have electrical filters that prevent visualization of the spikes unless special circuitry is turned on.

Step 3: Place a magnet over the device during ECG monitoring
- If asynchronous pacing at the expected battery rate is then observed, the device (a) is not an ICD and (b) the battery has adequate remaining charge.
- As batteries become depleted, the magnet rate drops at least 10 bpm below the normal battery rate (see Table 12.2 for specific normal values).
- The presence of a weak battery should be a trigger for expert involvement before proceeding to surgery for anything other than the most dire circumstances.

Step 4: Check electrolytes
- Patients on diuretics or acutely ill should have their electrolytes checked. Pacing thresholds can be affected by electrolyte disturbances.

Step 5: Contact a qualified individual
- This step should be performed whenever possible. This could be the person who normally manages the device or someone within your system.
- With your knowledge of the device and proposed surgery, it can be determined if interrogation is needed prior to surgery and which option is best (do nothing, place magnet, reprogram for surgery).

INTRAOPERATIVE MANAGEMENT

For all patients, the following management points should be employed:
- The cautery grounding pad should be located on the patient such that the cautery current is directed away from the device and leads.
- Some form of pulse monitor must be used during cautery. The pulse oximeter, routinely used during surgery, is adequate for this purpose.
- Recommendations for the use of bipolar cautery or short cautery bursts are almost always impractical and should be left to the OR personnel.
- Depending on the proximity of the cautery to the device and leads, patients dependent on the device to maintain a reasonable heart rate will typically be changed to asynchronous pacing. Magnet use on pacemakers will prevent bradycardia/asystole, but the high heart rate associated with the magnet use may not be appropriate for all patients.

- A discussion about the device settings between the programmer and the anesthesia team is helpful as the anesthesia team can contribute to the decision making process and be better aware of how the device might perform during surgery.
- The worst-case scenario is a patient with an ICD and pacemaker dependency having surgery above the umbilicus. The use of a magnet may prevent inadvertent shocks, but nothing can be done to prevent the cautery EMI from inhibiting the demand pacing. Should demand pacing be inhibited and the patient develops an inadequate pulse or asystole, then cautery bursts will have to be of limited duration.

IMPLANTABLE CARDIOVERTER-DEFIBRILLATOR MANAGEMENT
- Tachycardia sensing should be disabled to prevent unwanted shocks.
- If a magnet is used, the operator needs to know what feedback the device will provide (if any) to indicate that the device has sensed the magnet. In the event of an intraoperative tachyarrhythmia, simple removal of the magnet will reactivate the device.
- If tachy therapy is programmed off, then continuous ECG monitoring must be employed and an external defibrillator immediately available until tachy therapy is restored [7].

POSTOPERATIVE MANAGEMENT

Device interrogation after surgery should be performed [1]:
- To restore the original device settings.
- To make sure that the EMI has not caused any damage to the device or leads or resulted in a return to default settings. This is primarily a concern only when monopolar cautery was applied close to the device or leads.

Other situations which should prompt interrogation include the following:
- Cardioversion/defibrillation was performed.
- The patient had serious hemodynamic problems intraoperatively (such as chest compressions, massive bleeding, prolonged hypotension).
- The patient had radiofrequency ablation.

- A central line was placed.
- There were concerns about device function in the operating room.

Patients who were exposed to monopolar cautery below the umbilicus, had lithotripsy or electroconvulsive therapy, and did not need interrogation after the procedure should see their cardiologist within one month.

REFERENCES

1. Crossley GH, Poole JE, Rozner MA, Asirvatham SJ, Cheng A, Chung MK, Ferguson Jr TB, Gallagher JD, Gold MR, Hoyt RH, Irefin S, Kusumoto FM, Moorman LP, Thompson A. The Heart Rhythm Society Expert Consensus Statement on the perioperative management of patients with implantable defibrillators, pacemakers and arrhythmia monitors: facilities and patient management. Heart Rhythm. 2011;8:1114.
2. Allen M. Pacemakers and implantable cardioverter defibrillators. Anaesthesia. 2006;61: 883–90.
3. Moses HW, Mullin JC. A practical guide to cardiac pacing. 6th ed. Philadelphia, PA: Lippincott Williams & Wilkins; 2007. ISBN 978-0-7817-8881-6.
4. Bernstein AD, Daubert JC, Fletcher RD, et al. The revised NASPE/BPEG generic code for antibradycardia, adaptive-rate, and multisite pacing. Pacing Clin Electrophysiol. 2002;25: 260–4.
5. Leung S-K, Lau C-P. Developments in sensor-driven pacing. Cardiol Clin. 2000;18:113–55.
6. ASA task force on perioperative management of patients with cardiac implantable electronic devices. Practice advisory for the perioperative management of patients with cardiac implantable electronic devices: pacemakers and implantable cardioverter-defibrillators. Anesthesiology. 2011;114:247–61.
7. Fleisher LA, Fleischmann KE, Auerbach AD, et al. 2014 ACC/AHA guideline on perioperative cardiovascular evaluation and management of patients undergoing noncardiac surgery. J Am Coll Cardiol. 2014. doi: 10.1016/j.jacc.2014.07.944.
8. Schulman PM, Rozner MA. Use caution when applying magnets to pacemakers or defibrillators for surgery. Anesth Analg. 2013;117:422–7.
9. Rooke GA, Bowdle TA. Perioperative management of pacemakers and implantable cardioverter defibrillators: It's not just about the magnet (editorial). Anesth Analg. 2013;117:292–4.

Chapter 13
Diabetes Mellitus

Nason P. Hamlin and Kara J. Mitchell

BACKGROUND

Perioperative hyperglycemia increases the risk of infection and other complications. Perioperative control of hyperglycemia with insulin has been shown to nullify this increase even in patients not previously diagnosed as having diabetes [1–9]. Basal insulin therapy is key to good control, so think in terms of BASAL, BOLUS, and CORRECTION insulin (B-B-C), as shown in Table 13.1. The traditional practice of using only a "sliding scale" for insulin therapy should be abandoned [10].

PREOPERATIVE EVALUATION

Note the duration of the diabetes, the presence of complications (especially kidney disease), current management, and quality of glycemic control. An elevated HbA1c has been associated with worse surgical outcomes in observational and small prospective trials [11]; however, evidence to validate its use as a predictor of outcomes is lacking. Bariatric patients, for example, may only be able to achieve good glycemic control after surgery, so denying them surgery on the basis of an elevated HbA1c may not be optimal management. (Note: The HbA1c may be inaccurate due to end-stage renal disease, erythropoietin therapy, acute anemia, RBC transfusions, hemoglobinopathies, microhemolysis from heart valve replacement, increased RBC mass from testosterone therapy, HIV/AIDS, etc. [12]).

M.B. Jackson et al. (eds.), *The Perioperative Medicine Consult Handbook*, DOI 10.1007/978-3-319-09366-6_13,
© Springer International Publishing Switzerland 2015

TABLE 13.1 INSULIN TERMINOLOGY

BASAL insulin	Longer-acting insulins (e.g., glargine, detemir, and NPH) which provide a constant supply of "background" insulin, regardless of meals. All patients with type 1 diabetes *require* this and many with type 2 diabetes *need* this, especially in the perioperative period
BOLUS (prandial/ mealtime) insulin	The fixed dose (or altered dose for larger or smaller meals) of rapid-acting insulin (e.g., lispro, aspart, glulisine, or regular) which is given before a meal to mimic the body's normal response to a caloric load
CORRECTION insulin (replaces the older term "sliding scale")	The variable amount of rapid-acting insulin given *in addition to* the prandial and/or basal insulin to correct hyperglycemia. Correction insulin can also be given at bedtime although it is reasonable to be more conservative at this time due to the greater risk of nocturnal hypoglycemia

PERIOPERATIVE MANAGEMENT

FOR PROCEDURES THAT REQUIRE A RESTRICTED CALORIC INTAKE

For outpatient procedures, patients usually can resume home insulin, oral diabetes medication, and non-insulin injectable medication after the procedure, if they are eating. The following is applicable for patients who are to be NPO at midnight and are likely to have decreased caloric intake postoperatively:

- Hold bolus insulin the morning of surgery. Continue basal insulin the night before and the morning of surgery, but reduce the dose per Table 13.2.
- No oral hypoglycemic or non-insulin injectable meds the morning of surgery.
- In the recovery room/postanesthesia care unit, review the hyperglycemia plan for adequate insulin orders (see below for detailed recommendations).
- American Diabetes Association/American Association of Clinical Endocrinologists (ADA/AACE) guidelines recommend

TABLE 13.2 PREOPERATIVE INSULIN RECOMMENDATIONS

Basal insulin	*NPH (has a peak, thus provides some prandial coverage)*	75 % of the usual evening dose the night before surgery (no less than 80 % for type 1 DM) 50 % of the usual AM dose (if applicable) on the morning of surgery (80 % for type 1 DM)
	Glargine	Take 50–75 % of the usual evening dose (50 % if the patient takes more than 50 units, no less than 80 % for type 1 DM)
	Detemir	Take 50–75 % of the usual morning dose (50 % if the patient takes more than 50 units normally but no less than 80 % for type 1 DM)
	Premixed insulin (NPH/regular 70/30, Humalog® 75/25 or 50/50 mix, NovoLog® 70/30 mix)	Take 75 % of the usual evening dose (80 % type 1) Take 50 % of the usual morning dose (80 % type 1)
	Insulin pump	In general, continue basal rate, then switch to D5NS and an insulin infusion just prior to surgery, and disconnect the pump. Continue IV insulin until tolerating an adequate diet, and then resume the SC pump if the patient is stable, alert, and able to manage the pump. Endocrinology consultation should be considered
Bolus/prandial (mealtime) insulin	*Short-acting insulin*	Do not take on the morning of surgery with the exception of correction algorithms for hyperglycemia using rapid-acting analogues—lispro, aspart, or glulisine Note: Do not use regular insulin (U-100 and U-500) for correction due to prolonged duration of effect

managing non-insulin-requiring type 2 patients with insulin and not resuming oral diabetes medication and non-insulin injectable medication until the patient is ready to go home [6].

- If the patient has an insulin pump or continuous glucose monitor, consider recommending an endocrinology consultation.

USING AN INSTITUTIONAL INFUSION PROTOCOL AND TRANSITIONING TO SC INSULIN

- Start protocol when the patient presents to the preoperative holding area.
- Continue the insulin infusion until the patient is likely to be eating ~50 % of meals and has a reasonably stable blood sugar on the insulin infusion (see Table 13.3 to calculate the dose).
- If the patient normally takes basal insulin (e.g., glargine) in the morning, give the basal and bolus insulin before breakfast and stop the insulin infusion.
- If the patient normally takes basal insulin (e.g., glargine) at night and is starting to eat in the morning, give a one-time dose of NPH (roughly half the dose of the planned evening glargine) in the morning along with the short-acting bolus to serve as a bridge to the first glargine dose that evening.
- For patients transitioning at bedtime, continue the infusion for 2 h after the glargine, detemir, or NPH dose to compensate for the slower onset of the basal insulin (as bolus insulin is not usually scheduled at bedtime).
- Patients who are not eating, but who have had good glycemic control on a stable dose of insulin on the infusion for some time, may be transitioned to SC insulin calculating a basal insulin dose 60–80 % of the 24-h IV requirement plus q6h correction (but no prandial bolus) insulin.

NO INSTITUTIONAL INSULIN INFUSION PROTOCOL AVAILABLE

- Devise a subcutaneous basal and correction insulin plan for use while the patient is NPO.
- Add bolus insulin when the patient is eating: Cut the basal insulin dose in half and calculate the other half as bolus insulin divided equally before each meal, if meals are of similar size.
- Evaluate the blood glucose pattern for hyper- or hypoglycemia to determine which insulin should be adjusted.

TABLE 13.3 TRANSITIONING FROM IV TO SC INSULIN: CALCULATING THE DOSE

Guidelines

– The subcutaneous (SC) dose is only 60–80 % of the IV dose
– Post-op insulin requirements also tend to go down with time, so a reasonable plan is to calculate the amount of insulin given via infusion over the last 16 h to give you the estimated 24-h subcutaneous insulin requirement. Thus, the last 16-h total IV dose = next 24-h total SC dose
– Next, divide the 24-h SC dose into basal and prandial/premeal bolus[a,b]:
  – ~ 50 % of the estimated requirement is given as basal glargine, usually at bedtime, or NPH or detemir BID
  – ~ 50 % of the estimated requirement is given as lispro, aspart, or glulisine as three equally divided mealtime (prandial) doses

Example

Your patient has required 3 units of insulin IV per hour for the last 16 h
1. Calculate SC dose: 3 × 16 = 48 units total SC dose
2. Divide into basal and prandial:
  – Basal: ½ × 48 = 24 units of basal insulin (e.g., glargine qhs)
  – Prandial: ½ × 48 = 24 units of prandial insulin (e.g., lispro, aspart, or glulisine) divided before each meal. Thus, 24 units/3 = 8 units before each meal (if isocaloric)

[a]If the patient is not eating three full meals a day, you may want to give more than 50 % basal and less prandial insulin. If not eating at all, give 60–70 % as basal plus q6h correction insulin

[b]Modify the insulin dose by 20–30 % every day until the patient has optimal glycemic control. Although some concerns have been raised about "intensive" insulin therapy in the critical care setting [13–17], current guidelines target a premeal glucose <140 mg/dL and a random glucose <180 mg/dL (while avoiding hypoglycemia) for a majority of hospitalized patients who are not critically ill [18]

SPECIAL CONSIDERATIONS

- Gastric bypass and sleeve gastrectomy patients usually have a dramatic drop in insulin requirement starting the day after surgery, so the insulin dose needs to be reduced accordingly. Resuming metformin (if renal function is acceptable) at discharge is acceptable [19]. Insulin secretagogues (e.g., glipizide) are usually held.
- If the patient is on steroids, give no more than 40 % basal and at least 60 % prandial.

TABLE 13.4 ONSET, PEAK, AND DURATION OF EFFECT OF VARIOUS INSULINS

	Onset	Peak	Duration	Notes
Glargine	1 h	None	20–24 h	Typically dosed once daily but some require twice daily, especially in type 1 DM
Detemir	1 h	None	Variable; up to 23 h	Similar to glargine
NPH	1–1.5 h	4–12 h	Up to 24 h, usually 18–20 h	Rarely provides sufficient effect to allow for once daily dosing (typically dosed 2–3 times per day)
Lispro/aspart/glulisine	5–10 min	0.5–1.5 h	3–5 h	Residual effect can be seen out to 6–8 h. Prone to "stacking" with frequent correction doses
Regular	30–60 min	2–4 h	8–12 h	Should not be used as a correction dose. Use a rapid-acting analogue instead
U-500[a]				See below

[a]U-500 insulin use entails some special concerns. It is used in OB patients, patients with lipodystrophy, very insulin-resistant obese patients, and some others. If a patient was on U-500 at home, it is suggested that an endocrinologist be involved. The diabetes teaching team should also work with the patient's nurse

- Prandial (rapid-acting) insulin works best if given at least 10–15 min before the meal as this prevents large postprandial spikes. In the hospital this is not always possible but should be considered when titrating insulin doses, especially if the timing of the insulin changes frequently.
- The onset of regular insulin is 30–60 min. Consider using regular insulin for prandial coverage (but not correction dose) for patients with gastroparesis (but give closer to meal) or patients with chronic nausea, such as those receiving chemotherapy.
- See Table 13.4 for the onset, peak, and duration of effect of various insulins.

INSULIN MANAGEMENT WITH TPN AND TUBE FEEDING
Total Parenteral Nutrition
Use the insulin infusion rate to take a lot of the guesswork out of calculating the correct dose. For patients on TPN:

- Do not add insulin to the TPN bag until the patient is stable and the insulin requirement has been established using the insulin infusion protocol. Calculate the insulin requirement by adding up the number of units of insulin the patient received via the IV protocol for the previous 12 h and multiply by 2 for the 24-h requirement.
- Add 80–100 % of the calculated 24-h dose of insulin to the next night's TPN bag. Stop the insulin infusion when the insulin-containing TPN bag is started. Exception: See below for cyclic TPN. Correct with the subcutaneous insulin correction algorithm for hyperglycemia q 6 h. Choose the algorithm based on the total amount of insulin required (<40 units = low dose, 40–80 units = medium dose, >80 units = high dose). Adjust the amount of insulin in the TPN daily until the patient has adequate glycemic control (BG 140–180).
- If the patient is on cyclic TPN, make sure to use the insulin infusion rate during the time the TPN is running to calculate the amount of insulin to be added to the TPN bag. The patient may still need basal insulin while TPN is not running, either with NPH or via resumption of the insulin infusion during those hours. If the patient is eating while TPN is not running, prandial SC insulin may also be needed.

Tube Feeding
Recommendations for patients receiving tube feeds are shown in Table 13.5.

TABLE 13.5 INSULIN MANAGEMENT FOR PATIENTS RECEIVING TUBE FEEDS

Continuous tube feeds	■ Continue the insulin infusion protocol ■ If changing to subcutaneous insulin, use the insulin infusion requirement to calculate the dose, as described above, and then divide the short-acting (prandial) component into q6h doses of *regular* insulin ■ If the patient has not been on an insulin infusion, calculate the SC daily basal/prandial insulin requirement using body weight, 0.2–0.5 units/kg. Age, renal function, and baseline glucose control need to be considered in dosing
Bolus tube feeds	■ Give regular insulin 30–45 min before the bolus feed and check finger stick glucose 2 h later ■ Adjust the dose of insulin to achieve post-bolus target glucose of 140–180
Cyclic tube feeds[a]	■ 8-h cycle: Give $\frac{1}{3}$ to $\frac{1}{2}$ of the basal requirement as NPH and half as many units of the bolus dose as regular at the start of the cycle. Re-dose basal as needed 12 h after the initial dose ■ 12-h cycle: Give ½ the basal requirement as NPH and ¼ of the bolus requirement as regular at the start of the cycle and re-dose the regular insulin 6 h into the feed. Re-dose the basal as needed 12 h after the initial dose ■ Titrate the insulin dose daily until you achieve adequate glycemic control (BG 140–180) ■ The patient should also be corrected with a rapid-acting insulin algorithm for hyperglycemia q4h rather than premeal. Choose an algorithm based on the total amount of insulin required (i.e., <40 units = low dose, 40–80 units = medium dose, >80 units = high dose)

[a]Note: Cyclic tube feeds are challenging. Covering an 8–12-h "meal" followed by 16–12 h of "fasting" requires constant titration of insulin doses based on glucose monitoring. Tube feeds may also be interrupted by procedures or clogging of the tube, thus increasing the risk for hypoglycemia

REFERENCES

1. Frisch A, et al. Prevalence and clinical outcome of hyperglycemia in the perioperative period in noncardiac surgery. Diabetes Care. 2010;33:1783–8.
2. Pomposelli JJ, Baxter JK, Babineau TJ, et al. Early postoperative glucose control predicts nosocomial infection rate in diabetic patients. J Parenter Enteral Nutr. 1998;22(2):77–81.
3. Dellinger EP. Preventing surgical-site infections: the importance of timing and glucose control. Infect Control Hosp Epidemiol. 2001;22:604–6.
4. Inzucchi SE. Management of hyperglycemia in the hospital setting. N Engl J Med. 2006;355(18):1903–11.

5. Ramos M, et al. Relationship of perioperative hyperglycemia and postoperative infections in patients who undergo general and vascular surgery. Ann Surg. 2008;248:585–91.
6. Moghissi ES, Korytkowski MT, DiNardo M, et al. American Association of Clinical Endocrinologists and American Diabetes Association consensus statement on inpatient glycemic control. Endocrinol Pract. 2009;15(4):1–17.
7. Kwon S, Thompson R, Dellinger P, et al. Importance of perioperative glycemic control in general surgery. Ann Surg. 2013;257(1):8–14.
8. Umpierrez GE, Smiley D, Jacobs S, et al. Randomized Study of Basal-Bolus Insulin Therapy in the inpatient management of patients with Type 2 diabetes undergoing general surgery (RABBIT 2 surgery). Diabetes Care. 2011;34:256–61.
9. Kiran RP, Turina M, Hammel J, et al. The clinical significance of an elevated postoperative glucose value in nondiabetic patients after colorectal surgery. Ann Surg. 2013;258(4):599605.
10. Hirsch IB. Sliding scale insulin-time to stop sliding. JAMA. 2009;301(2):213–4.
11. Perna M, Romagnuolo J, Morgan K, et al. Preoperative hemoglobinA1c and postoperative glucose control in outcomes after gastric bypass for obesity. Surg Obesity Rel Dis. 2012; 8(6):685–90.
12. Wright LAC, Hirsch IB. The challenge of the use of glycemic biomarkers in diabetes: Reflecting on hemoglobin A1C, 1,5-anhydroglucitol, and the glycated proteins fructosamine and albumin. Diabetes Spectrum. 2012;25:141–8.
13. The NICE-Study Investigators. Intensive versus conventional glucose control in critically ill patients. N Engl J Med. 2009;360(13):1283–97.
14. Inzucchi SE, Siegle MD. Glucose control in the ICU—how tight is too tight? N Engl J Med. 2009;360(13):1346–9.
15. Griesdale DE, de Souza RJ, van Dam RM, et al. Intensive insulin therapy and mortality among critically ill patients: a meta-analysis including the NICE-SUGAR study data. CMAJ. 2009;180(8):821–7.
16. Joint Statement from ADA and AACE on the NICE-SUGAR study on intensive versus conventional glucose control in critically ill patients. https://www.aace.com/files/inpatientglycemic-controlconsensusstatement.pdf. Accessed 22 Oct 2014.
17. Kasangara D, et al. Intensive insulin therapy in hospitalized patients: a systematic review. Ann Intern Med. 2011;154:268–82.
18. Umpierrez GE, Hellman R, Korytkowski MT, Kosiborod M, Maynard GA, Montori VM, Seley JJ, Van den Berghe G. Endocrine society. Management of hyperglycemia in hospitalized patients in non-critical care setting: an endocrine society clinical practice guideline. J Clin Endocrinol Metab. 2012;97(1):16–38.
19. Lipska KJ, et al. Use of metformin in the setting of mild to moderate renal insufficiency. Diabetes Care. 2011;34(6):1431–7.

Chapter 14
Stress-Dose Steroids

Kara J. Mitchell

BACKGROUND

Patients are treated with glucocorticoids for a multitude of conditions, including chronic obstructive pulmonary disease (COPD), organ transplantation, autoimmune diseases, and other inflammatory states. This chapter addresses supplemental steroid dosing (commonly called "stress-dose steroids") for patients with tertiary (iatrogenic) adrenal insufficiency as a result of glucocorticoid (GC) use. The use of supplemental perioperative steroids in patients with adrenal insufficiency is controversial [1].

PREOPERATIVE EVALUATION

First, assess whether the patient's hypothalamic-pituitary-adrenal (HPA) IS suppressed, MAY BE suppressed, or is NOT suppressed:

- Higher doses and longer duration of GC therapy render the axis more suppressed, but considerable variability is seen between patients [2, 3, 5]; see Table 14.1.
- Recovery from tertiary adrenal insufficiency may take months [2, 5], so the clinical history should include all GC use within the past year.
- All patients with primary adrenal insufficiency (Addison's disease) or ACTH deficiency (hypothalamic/pituitary dysfunction) have inadequate GC production [2].

M.B. Jackson et al. (eds.), *The Perioperative Medicine Consult Handbook*, DOI 10.1007/978-3-319-09366-6_14,
© Springer International Publishing Switzerland 2015

TABLE 14.1 HPA AXIS SUPPRESSION BASED ON GLUCOCORTICOID EXPOSURE HISTORY [3]

HPA axis status	Glucocorticoid (GC) exposure	Management
NOT suppressed	■ <3 weeks ■ Every-other-day therapy ■ AM dose of <5 mg prednisone or equivalent[a]	Take usual AM dose of GC
MAY be suppressed	■ Intermediate-dose GC use (5–20 mg prednisone or equivalent/day) ■ Inhaled GC use ■ >3 GC intra-articular or spinal injections in the past 3 months ■ Class I topical GC use[b] ■ Significant GC use in the past year	Check 8 AM serum cortisol (24 h off usual GC dose) vs. empiric supplemental GC without testing ■ If <5mcg/dL, supplemental GC ■ If >10mcg/dL, take usual AM dose of GC ■ If 5–10mcg/dL, do ACTH stimulation test [4] vs. empiric supplemental GC
IS suppressed	■ >20 mg/day of prednisone or equivalent for >3 weeks ■ Clinically Cushingoid appearance[c]	Supplemental GC

[a]5 mg prednisone = 4 mg methylprednisolone = 0.75 mg dexamethasone = 20 mg hydrocortisone
[b]Class I topical glucocorticoids include betamethasone dipropionate 0.05 %, clobetasol propionate 0.05 %, diflorasone diacetate 0.05 %, fluocinonide 0.1 %, and halobetasol propionate 0.05 %
[c]Prominent central obesity, "moon" facies, dorsocervical fat pad, and/or bulging supraclavicular fat pads

PERIOPERATIVE MANAGEMENT

If you decide that supplemental dose steroids are indicated for a patient, use Table 14.2 to find the recommended dose. These recommendations are based on expert opinion, as only two small prospective trials on this topic exist [1, 6]. Consider:
- The patient's preoperative GC dose
- Anticipated duration and stress of surgery
- Concomitant use of medications (i.e., rifampin) that alter GC metabolism
- Possible complications of steroid administration (see Table 14.3)

TABLE 14.2 DOSING FOR SUPPLEMENTAL GLUCOCORTICOID ADMINIS-
TRATION [6]

Surgical risk	Examples	Recommendation
Minor surgery	Inguinal hernia repair Colonoscopy	Take usual AM steroid dose
Moderate surgery	Open cholecystectomy Total knee replacement Abdominal hysterectomy	Take usual AM steroid dose plus 25–50 mg hydrocortisone IV prior to surgery followed by 50–75 mg hydrocortisone equivalent $\times$ 1–2 days (e.g., 25 mg q 8 h $\times$ 24 h); then resume baseline dose[a]
Major surgery	Whipple Esophagectomy Total proctocolectomy Cardiac surgery	Take usual AM steroid dose plus 25–100 mg hydrocortisone prior to surgery followed by 100–150 mg of hydrocortisone equivalent per day for 2–3 days (e.g., 50 mg q 8 h $\times$ 48 h); then taper dose by 1/2 per day until maintenance dose is reached[b]

[a]The exact dosing may be tailored to take into account the patient's baseline corticosteroid dose. In some cases, the baseline dose exceeds stress dosages, and continuing the baseline dose is reasonable
[b]For very long surgeries, some advocate giving additional doses intraoperatively, or using dexamethasone. Also, if surgical complications are encountered postoperatively, a longer duration of supplemental steroid administration may be indicated

TABLE 14.3 COMPLICATIONS OF GLUCOCORTICOID THERAPY

HPA axis suppression
Impaired wound healing
Skin thinning and easy bruising
Reduced bone mass, leading to fracture
Increased susceptibility to infections
Insomnia, mania, psychosis
Ulcer/gastrointestinal bleeding
Insulin resistance
Fluid retention/worsened blood pressure control
Subcapsular cataract formation
Myopathy/proximal muscle weakness

Patients receiving GC therapy should be followed clinically for complications, such as those noted in Table 14.3 [2, 3, 5, 6].

REFERENCES

1. Yong SL, Marik P, Esposito M, Coulthard P. Supplemental perioperative steroids for surgical patients with adrenal insufficiency. Cochrane Database Syst Rev 2009; 7:CD005367 [Note that a subsequent review (Cochrane Database Syst Rev 2012; 12:CD005367) has been withdrawn from publication as of 10/17/2013, due to "correspondence which have challenged the eligibility criteria and interpretation of the evidence summarized."]
2. Lamberts SW, Bruining HA, deJong FH. Corticosteroid therapy in severe illness. N Engl J Med. 1997;337:1285–92.
3. Hamrahian AH, Sanziana R, Milan S. The surgical patient taking glucocorticoids. In: Basow DS, editor. UpToDate. Waltham, MA; 2014. Accessed 11 Jan 2014
4. Dorin RI, Qualls CR, Crapo LM. Diagnosis of adrenal insufficiency. Ann Intern Med. 2003;139(3):194–204.
5. Coursin DB, Wood KE. Corticosteroid supplementation for adrenal insufficiency. JAMA. 2002;287(2):236–40.
6. Salem M, Tainsh RE, Bromberg J, et al. Perioperative glucocorticoid coverage: a reassessment 42 years after emergence of a problem. Ann Surg. 1994;219:416–25.

Chapter 15
Thyroid Disease

Jennifer R. Lyden and Jeanie C. Yoon

BACKGROUND

Disorders of the thyroid gland are common. Millions of Americans are living with subclinical or overt thyroid dysfunction [1–3], and physicians who provide perioperative care are frequently asked to assess surgical risk and assist in the management of patients with thyroid disease.

Thyroid hormone affects virtually every organ system in the body [1]. In the perioperative period, the effects of thyroid imbalance range from clinically insignificant to shock and catastrophic multiorgan system failure [4]. Despite the prevalence of thyroid dysfunction and its potential impact on surgical patients, there is a paucity of data examining surgical outcomes in those with thyroid disease.

PREOPERATIVE EVALUATION

PATIENTS NOT KNOWN TO HAVE THYROID DYSFUNCTION

There is no evidence to support routine preoperative thyroid testing in asymptomatic patients. Consider screening for thyroid disease with a serum TSH if there is a clinical concern for new or poorly controlled thyroid disease. Signs and symptoms of thyroid dysfunction include:

- Hypothyroidism: weight gain, lethargy, fatigue, cold intolerance, anorexia, dry skin, and brittle hair.
- Hyperthyroidism: tachycardia, atrial fibrillation, fever, weight loss, tremor, goiter, and ophthalmopathy.

M.B. Jackson et al. (eds.), *The Perioperative Medicine Consult Handbook*, DOI 10.1007/978-3-319-09366-6_15,
© Springer International Publishing Switzerland 2015

PATIENTS WITH KNOWN HYPOTHYROIDISM

- Patients with stable disease (e.g., no recent medication changes and recently documented euthyroid state) do not require screening TSH preoperatively.
- Newly diagnosed patients, those with recent changes to hormone replacement therapy, or those with history and/or physical examination that suggests thyroid hormone imbalance should have screening TSH preoperatively.
- Consider preoperative screening TSH in hypothyroid patients treated with animal-derived desiccated thyroid preparations (e.g., Armour Thyroid®, Nature-Throid®) given greater risk of product variability and lack of evidence to guide its use [5].

PATIENTS WITH KNOWN HYPERTHYROIDISM

- Consider checking baseline thyroid function tests (TSH and free T4), CBC with differential and liver enzymes (to evaluate for efficacy and toxicity of antithyroid medication) in all hyperthyroid patients if not done within the last 3–6 months.
- Newly diagnosed patients, those with recent medication changes, or those with history and/or physical examination that suggests thyroid hormone imbalance should have thyroid function tests (TSH and free T4) preoperatively. Consider adding a total T3 if TSH is suppressed and there is concern for thyrotoxicosis.
- Assess for changes in thyroid size/shape which might affect the patient's airway; inform anesthesiologist if concerned.

PERIOPERATIVE MANAGEMENT

HYPOTHYROIDISM

Patients with treated hypothyroidism should continue thyroid hormone replacement therapy in the perioperative period including the morning of surgery and postoperatively:

- If oral access is unavailable, hormone replacement can be held safely for 6–7 days given its long half-life [6]; it can also be given parenterally (usually at half the oral dose).
- Patients receiving thyroid hormone replacement via feeding tube with or without concurrent enteral nutrition are at risk of developing subclinical or overt hypothyroidism [7, 8].
- There are no data to suggest empiric dose adjustments or holding enteral nutrition pre- and post administration of thyroid hormone is beneficial [7, 8].

TABLE 15.1 PERIOPERATIVE MANAGEMENT OF PATIENTS WITH HYPOTHYROIDISM

Degree of thyroid dysfunction	Laboratory findings	Elective	Urgent/ emergent	Treatment
Subclinical	■ Increased TSH ■ Normal free T4	■ Proceed	■ Proceed	■ None
Mild–moderate	■ Increased TSH ■ Low free T4	■ Delay	■ Proceed	■ Standard replacement (1.7mcg/kg PO Qday. Adjust dose q4–6weeks based on TFTs)
Severe	■ Myxedema coma[a] ■ Free T4 < 1ug/dL	■ Delay	■ Proceed	■ Endocrinology consultation ■ Emergent hormone replacement[b] ■ Hydrocortisone 100 mg IV Q8 h

[a]Myxedema coma is a medical emergency with a high mortality rate. Optimal management for myxedema coma is unclear [15] (see below)
[b]Initial T4 loading dose of 200–500 mcg ×1 followed by 50–100 mcg daily [16, 17]

- Consider monitoring TSH in patients on prolonged enteral nutrition.

There is little published data to help guide the management of hypothyroid patients perioperatively:

- No randomized trials have examined perioperative outcomes in euthyroid patients compared to those with thyroid dysfunction.
- Retrospective cohort studies have shown increased rates of complications associated with hypothyroid states [9].

Most experts agree that decisions to delay surgery be based on the degree of hypothyroidism and urgency of surgical intervention [10, 11]:

- In general, if time and clinical circumstances allow, achieving a euthyroid state prior to surgical intervention is optimal (Table 15.1) [11–13].
- Patients with subclinical hypothyroidism (elevated TSH, normal free T4 and T3) can typically proceed with elective surgeries.

TABLE 15.2 PERIOPERATIVE COMPLICATIONS IN PATIENTS WITH HYPOTHYROIDISM

Cardiovascular [3, 11, 12, 14]
- Decreased cardiac output from decreased heart rate and stroke volume contractility
- Decreased total blood volume from increased peripheral vascular resistance (increased mean arterial pressure suppresses the renin-angiotensin-aldosterone system which in turn decreases sodium absorption and blood volume)

Pulmonary [3, 11, 12, 14]
- Respiratory failure from decreased hypoxic and hypercapnic ventilatory drive
- Respiratory muscle weakness

Renal [3, 11, 12, 14]
- Decreased renal perfusion
- Inappropriate secretion of antidiuretic hormone leading to alterations in fluid and electrolyte balance
- Decreased renal clearance of medications/anesthesia

Gastrointestinal [3, 11, 12, 14]
- Delayed gastric emptying and gut motility

Metabolic [3, 11, 12, 14]
- Delayed metabolism leading to prolonged half-life of certain medications

Immunologic [3, 11, 14]
- Impaired ability to mount a febrile response

- If surgical intervention is necessary or emergent, surgeons, anesthetists, and internists should be aware that perioperative complications may occur in those with mild to moderate hypothyroidism [3, 11, 12, 14]. Close cardiovascular, respiratory, and renal monitoring is suggested (Table 15.2).

Thyroid Function in the Critically Ill [18–21]
Critical illness is associated with alterations in concentrations of thyroid hormones. Previously known as "euthyroid sick syndrome," this syndrome is now termed "non-thyroidal illness." Laboratory data suggests transient central hypothyroidism:
- T3 usually low
- T4 and free T4 low or normal
- TSH low or normal

The degree of illness generally correlates with the degree of thyroid hormone abnormalities. There is no evidence that thyroid hormone replacement is beneficial and may be harmful. Thyroid function should not be checked in critically ill patients unless there is strong suspicion and/or clinical evidence of thyroid dysfunction (e.g., bradycardia, hypothermia, altered mental status, etc.).

The Hypothyroid Patient Undergoing Cardiovascular Surgery
- Thyroid hormone has profound effects on the cardiovascular system [22], but replacement is controversial in cardiac surgeries.
- Replacement may precipitate acute coronary syndromes.
- Untreated hypothyroidism may precipitate or exacerbate heart failure and/or hypotension in the perioperative period.
- Minimal data available, but prior studies suggest no adverse events in mild to moderate hypothyroidism when hormone replacement deferred [23, 24].
- Decision to initiate thyroid hormone replacement should be made based on the degree of hormone imbalance, severity of heart failure, and hemodynamic instability.

Myxedema Coma
In rare cases, the stress of surgery can trigger myxedema coma in patients with hypothyroidism: severe hypothyroidism representing a medical emergency with a high mortality rate [3, 15, 25]. The clinical presentation of myxedema coma includes:
- Decreased level of consciousness
- Hypothermia
- Cardiovascular effects: hypotension, bradycardia, and cardiac arrhythmias
- Hypoventilation
- Hyponatremia
- Hypoglycemia [14]

The diagnosis is based on a high TSH, very low free T4, and the clinical presentation. If myxedema coma is suspected, cortisol and cosyntropin stimulation test should be sent if possible to assess for associated adrenal insufficiency or hypopituitarism. Treatment usually requires intensive supportive measures, depending on the severity of hypothyroidism [16]:
- Admission to intensive care unit
- Mechanical ventilation
- Rewarming
- Volume resuscitation and/or vasopressor support

- Cardiac monitoring
- Stress dose steroids until adrenal insufficiency excluded [15]

Hormone replacement should be initiated in any patient suspected of myxedema coma, in collaboration with a thyroid specialist. The exact hormone replacement regimen is controversial, [16, 17] but some useful guidelines include:

- IV preparations of T4 and T3 available; avoid oral replacement given unknown absorption [16].
- T3 has been associated with increased risk of cardiac ischemia and/or arrhythmias [26]; however, there are minimal data to support this [27, 28].
- Initial T4 loading dose of 200–500 mcg x1 followed by 50–100 mcg daily [16, 17].

HYPERTHYROIDISM
Non-thyroid Surgery

There are scant data evaluating the risk of hyperthyroidism in non-thyroid surgery. One small retrospective study in elderly patients undergoing surgical fixation for hip fractures found that overt hyperthyroidism on admission was associated with an increased risk for 30-day postoperative complications. [29] In addition, hyperthyroidism has significant cardiopulmonary effects that may increase the risk of surgery [30, 31] (see Table 15.3). Care should usually be coordinated with a thyroid specialist, but general principles include:

- Patients with known hyperthyroidism should continue hyperthyroid medications throughout the perioperative period including the morning of surgery.
- Elective surgery should be postponed in patients with poorly controlled or untreated hyperthyroidism until they are euthyroid, due to the risk of thyroid storm (see Table 15.4).
- Patients should be treated with an antithyroid medication prior to nonurgent surgery until they are euthyroid.
- Patients with subclinical hyperthyroidism (low TSH, normal free T4 and T3) can typically proceed with elective surgeries.
- Subclinical hyperthyroidism has been associated with increased risk of atrial fibrillation in older patients [32, 33]. Consider perioperative beta-blockade in older patients (>50 years) or younger patients with cardiovascular disease, and taper after recovery.

Thyroid Surgery

In general, care should be coordinated with a thyroid specialist. Studies suggest that perioperative beta-blockers alone effectively con-

TABLE 15.3 PERIOPERATIVE COMPLICATIONS IN PATIENTS WITH HYPERTHYROIDISM

Cardiovascular [35]
- Arrhythmias, e.g., atrial fibrillation [36]
- Tachycardia, systolic hypertension, widened pulse pressure from decreased peripheral vascular resistance
- Congestive heart failure
- Pulmonary hypertension [37, 38]
- Angina from increased myocardial oxygen demand

Pulmonary
- Dyspnea due to increased oxygen consumption and CO_2 production
- Respiratory and skeletal muscle weakness
- Decreased lung volume

Gastrointestinal
- Increased gut motility with malabsorption, malnutrition

Metabolic
- Increased basal metabolic rate

Psychiatric
- Delirium, psychosis, decreased mental status

TABLE 15.4 PERIOPERATIVE MANAGEMENT OF PATIENTS WITH HYPERTHYROIDISM

Degree of thyroid dysfunction	Laboratory findings	Elective	Urgent/ emergent	Treatment
Subclinical	- Low TSH - Normal free T4	Proceed	Proceed	- Consider beta-blockade for older patients (>50 years) or younger patients with cardio-vascular disease
Mild–moderate	- Low TSH - High free T4	Delay	Proceed	- Endocrinology consult - Beta-blockade (e.g., atenolol, metoprolol) for goal HR 60–80[a] - Thionamide (methima-zole preferred) - Inorganic iodide (e.g., SSKI) for Graves' disease

(continued)

TABLE 15.4 (CONTINUED)

Degree of thyroid dysfunction	Laboratory findings	Elective	Urgent/ emergent	Treatment
Severe	Severe clinical signs, thyroid storm	Delay	Proceed	■ ICU transfer ■ Endocrinology consult ■ High-dose thionamide (PTU or methimazole, oral or rectal), beta-blockade (propranolol, esmolol)[a], inorganic iodide (SSKI), and glucocorticoids (hydrocortisone, dexamethasone) [39]. Start treatment empirically while awaiting test results ■ Consider the use of iodinated radiocontrast agent, e.g., iopanoic acid if available[b] [40] ■ Supportive care: acetaminophen, cooling blankets, volume resuscitation, glycemic control ■ Workup for other precipitating causes (e.g., infection)

[a]Propranolol can be used intraoperatively [41]
[b]Iopanoic acid and ipodate are currently not available in the USA [42]

trol the clinical manifestations of hyperthyroidism and are as effective as thionamides with similar low rates of anesthetic and cardiovascular complications [34]. In thyroidectomy for Graves' disease, inorganic iodide can be used starting 10 days before to decrease thyroid vascularity and surgical blood loss. For post-thyroidectomy patients, the medicine consultant should be vigilant for:

■ Neck wound hemorrhage or infection
■ Vocal cord paralysis
■ Hypocalcemia (sign of hypoparathyroidism)
■ Symptoms of thyrotoxicosis

Thyroid Storm

The most serious perioperative complication associated with hyperthyroidism is thyroid storm. Thyroid storm is rare, usually occurs during surgery or within 18 h after surgery, and carries a high mortality, up to 40 % [43]. Diagnosis of thyroid storm is clinical: degree of TSH suppression or thyroid hormone elevation does not help differentiate between thyroid storm and uncomplicated hyperthyroidism. Signs include tachycardia, heart failure, hyperpyrexia, altered mental status, nausea, diarrhea, and hepatic failure. If thyroid storm is suspected, empiric treatment should be started promptly and workup initiated for precipitating causes (e.g., infection) while awaiting thyroid test results (see Table 15.4).

REFERENCES

1. Brent GA. Mechanisms of thyroid hormone action. J Clin Invest. 2012;122(9):3035–43.
2. Vanderpump MP. The epidemiology of thyroid disease. Br Med Bull. 2011;99:39–51.
3. Werner SC, Ingbar SH, Braverman LE, Utiger RD. Werner & Ingbar's the thyroid: a fundamental and clinical text. 9th ed. Philadelphia: Lippincott Williams & Wilkins; 2005.
4. Taylor PN, Razvi S, Pearce SH, Dayan CM. Clinical review: a review of the clinical consequences of variation in thyroid function within the reference range. J Clin Endocrinol Metab. 2013;98(9):3562–71.
5. Garber JR, Cobin RH, Gharib H, et al. Clinical practice guidelines for hypothyroidism in adults: cosponsored by the American Association of Clinical Endocrinologists and the American Thyroid Association. Endocr Pract. 2012;18(6):988–1028.
6. Schiff RL, Welsh GA. Perioperative evaluation and management of the patient with endocrine dysfunction. Med Clin North Am. 2003;87(1):175–92.
7. Dickerson RN, Maish 3rd GO, Minard G, Brown RO. Clinical relevancy of the levothyroxine-continuous enteral nutrition interaction. Nutr Clin Pract. 2010;25(6):646–52.
8. Manessis A, Lascher S, Bukberg P, et al. Quantifying amount of adsorption of levothyroxine by percutaneous endoscopic gastrostomy tubes. JPEN J Parenter Enteral Nutr. 2008; 32(2):197–200.
9. Weinberg AD, Brennan MD, Gorman CA, Marsh HM, O'Fallon WM. Outcome of anesthesia and surgery in hypothyroid patients. Arch Intern Med. 1983;143(5):893–7.
10. Gualandro DM, Pinho C, et al. I guidelines for perioperative evaluation. Arq Bras Cardiol. 2007;89(6):210–37.
11. Stathatos N, Wartofsky L. Perioperative management of patients with hypothyroidism. Endocrinol Metab Clin North Am. 2003;32(2):503–18.
12. Graham GW, Unger BP, Coursin DB. Perioperative management of selected endocrine disorders. Int Anesthesiol Clin. 2000;38(4):31–67.
13. Vanderpump MP, Tunbridge WM. Epidemiology and prevention of clinical and subclinical hypothyroidism. Thyroid. 2002;12(10):839–47.
14. Murkin JM. Anesthesia and hypothyroidism: a review of thyroxine physiology, pharmacology, and anesthetic implications. Anesth Analg. 1982;61(4):371–83.
15. Kwaku MP, Burman KD. Myxedema coma. J Intensive Care Med. 2007;22(4):224–31.
16. Klubo-Gwiezdzinska J, Wartofsky L. Thyroid emergencies. Med Clin North Am. 2012; 96(2):385–403.
17. Wall CR. Myxedema coma: diagnosis and treatment. Am Fam Physician. 2000;62(11):2485–90.
18. Stockigt JR. Guidelines for diagnosis and monitoring of thyroid disease: nonthyroidal illness. Clin Chem. 1996;42(1):188–92.
19. Wartofsky L, Burman KD. Alterations in thyroid function in patients with systemic illness: the "euthyroid sick syndrome". Endocr Rev. 1982;3(2):164–217.
20. DeGroot LJ. "Non-thyroidal illness syndrome" is functional central hypothyroidism, and if severe, hormone replacement is appropriate in light of present knowledge. J Endocrinol Invest. 2003;26(12):1163–70.

21. Adler SM, Wartofsky L. The nonthyroidal illness syndrome. Endocrinol Metab Clin North Am. 2007;36(3):657–672, vi.
22. Klein I, Danzi S. Thyroid disease and the heart. Circulation. 2007;116(15):1725–35.
23. Myerowitz PD, Kamienski RW, Swanson DK, et al. Diagnosis and management of the hypothyroid patient with chest pain. J Thorac Cardiovasc Surg. 1983;86(1):57–60.
24. Drucker DJ, Burrow GN. Cardiovascular surgery in the hypothyroid patient. Arch Intern Med. 1985;145(9):1585–7.
25. Arlot S, Debussche X, Lalau JD, et al. Myxoedema coma: response of thyroid hormones with oral and intravenous high-dose L-thyroxine treatment. Intensive Care Med. 1991;17(1): 16–8.
26. Yamamoto T, Fukuyama J, Fujiyoshi A. Factors associated with mortality of myxedema coma: report of eight cases and literature survey. Thyroid. 1999;9(12):1167–74.
27. Guden M, Akpinar B, Saggbas E, Sanisoglu I, Cakali E, Bayindir O. Effects of intravenous triiodothyronine during coronary artery bypass surgery. Asian Cardiovasc Thorac Ann. 2002;10(3):219–22.
28. Hamilton MA, Stevenson LW, Fonarow GC, et al. Safety and hemodynamic effects of intravenous triiodothyronine in advanced congestive heart failure. Am J Cardiol. 1998;81(4): 443–7.
29. Ling XW. ea. Preoperative thyroid dysfunction predicts 30-day postoperative complications in elderly patients with hip fracture. Geriatric Orthopaedic Surgery and Rehabilitation. Geriatric Orthopaedic Surgery and. Rehabilitation. 2013;4(2):43–9.
30. Klein IDS. Thyroid disease and the heart. Circulation. 2007;116(15):1725–35.
31. Sawin CT, et al. Low serum thyrotropic concentrations as a risk factor for atrial fibrillation in older persons. N Engl J Med. 1994;331:1249–52.
32. Sawin CTGA, Wolf PA, Belanger AJ, Baker E, Bacharach P, Wilson PW, Benjamin EJ, D'Agostino RB. Low serum thyrotropin concentrations as a risk factor for atrial fibrillation in older persons. N Engl J Med. 1994;331:1249–52.
33. Cappola ARFL, Arnold AM, Danese MD, Kuller LH, Burke GL, Tracy RP, Ladenson PW. Thyroid status, cardiovascular risk, and mortality in older adults. JAMA. 2006;2006(295): 1033–41.
34. Adlerberth ASG, Hasselgren PO. The selective beta 1-blocking agent metoprolol compared with antithyroid drug and thyroxine as preoperative treatment of patients with hyperthyroidism. Results from a prospective, randomized study. Ann Surg. 1987;205(2):182.
35. Ka W. Thyrotoxicosis and the heart. N Engl J Med. 1992;372(2):94.
36. Frost LVP, Mosekilde L. Hyperthyroidism and risk of atrial fibrillation or flutter: a population-based study. Arch Intern Med. 2004;164(15):1675.
37. Mercé JFS, Oltra C, Sanz E, Vendrell J, Simón I, Camprubí M, Bardají A, Ridao C. Cardiovascular abnormalities in hyperthyroidism: a prospective Doppler echocardiographic study. Am J Med. 2005;118(2):126.
38. Siu CW, Zhang XH, Yung C, Kung AW, Lau CP, Tse HF. Hemodynamic changes in hyperthyroidism-related pulmonary hypertension: a prospective echocardiographic study. J Clin Endocrinol Metab. 2007;92(5):1736.
39. Bahn Chair RS, Burch HB, Cooper DS, Garber JR, Greenlee MC, Klein I, Laurberg P, McDougall IR, Montori VM, Rivkees SA, Ross DS, Sosa JA, Stan MN, American Thyroid Association, American Association of Clinical Endocrinologists. Hyperthyroidism and other causes of thyrotoxicosis: management guidelines of the American Thyroid Association and American Association of Clinical Endocrinologists. Thyroid. 2011;21(6):593.
40. Panzer C, Beazley R, Braverman L. Rapid preoperative preparation for severe hyperthyroid Graves'. J Clin Endocrinol Metab. 2004;89(5):2142.
41. Das G, Krieger M. Treatment of thyrotoxic storm with intravenous administration of propranolol. Ann Intern Med. 1969;70(5):985.
42. Ross DS. Iodinated radiocontrast agents in the treatment of hyperthyroidism. UpToDate 2013.
43. Burch HBWL. Life-threatening thyrotoxicosis. Thyroid storm. Endocrinol Metab Clin North Am. 1993;22(2):263.

Chapter 16
Liver Disease and Perioperative Risk

Kara J. Mitchell

BACKGROUND

Acute hepatitis and cirrhosis are major risk factors for complications of surgery due to a number of physiologic changes [1, 2]:

- Baseline increased cardiac index and decreased systemic vascular resistance, augmented by anesthetics and blood loss
- Poor hepatic metabolism of anesthetic agents and other medications administered perioperatively and risk for hepatic encephalopathy
- Bleeding risk from impaired synthesis of thrombopoietin and clotting factors, splenic platelet sequestration, and portal hypertension-induced varices
- Pulmonary risk from ascites or pleural effusions (restriction); pulmonary hypertension and/or hepatopulmonary syndrome
- Infection risk due to impaired reticuloendothelial cell function and ascites-related risk for abdominal wound dehiscence
- Risk for renal insufficiency due to hypotension, ascites, diuretic therapy, and/or hepatorenal syndrome

Patients with compensated liver disease (mild chronic hepatitis, non-alcoholic fatty liver disease, etc.) generally tolerate surgery well [2, 3]. Patients with severe or decompensated liver disease, however, may have a mortality approaching 80 % [1, 2, 4]. The role of the medical consultant includes preoperative risk assessment, optimization of liver disease, and prevention and management of postoperative complications.

M.B. Jackson et al. (eds.), *The Perioperative Medicine Consult Handbook*, DOI 10.1007/978-3-319-09366-6_16,
© Springer International Publishing Switzerland 2015

PREOPERATIVE EVALUATION

ASYMPTOMATIC PATIENTS NOT KNOWN TO HAVE LIVER DISEASE

- Ask about: alcohol use, blood transfusions, IV drug use, and sexual history
- Look for: jaundice, spider telangiectasias, palmar erythema, gynecomastia, testicular atrophy, splenomegaly, encephalopathy, ascites, and peripheral edema
- Checking liver biochemical tests for screening purposes in asymptomatic patients is generally not recommended [2]

RISK STRATIFICATION OF PATIENTS WITH KNOWN OR SUSPECTED LIVER DISEASE

History and exam should be directed at the current state of the patient's liver disease, medication regimen, volume status, and prior history of complications, including response to previous surgeries or anesthesia. Surgeries that carry the highest risk for patients with liver disease include the following:

- Emergency and trauma surgery
- Surgery involving significant blood loss (>150 ml)
- Intra-abdominal surgery, especially if there has been previous abdominal surgery and lysis of vascular adhesions is required
- Hepatic resection

Hepatitis

Acute viral hepatitis carried a 10–13 % mortality in two studies of open liver biopsy between 1958 and 1963 [1, 2]. A similar study and a small case series of patients with alcoholic hepatitis demonstrated a 55–100 % mortality after laparotomy [1, 2]. Obese patients with non-alcoholic fatty liver disease (NAFLD) are not thought to be at increased risk for bariatric surgery, in the absence of portal hypertension or other independent risk factors [3].

Cirrhosis

Most experts recommend the use of both the Child-Turcotte-Pugh (CTP) classification and the Model for End-Stage Liver Disease (MELD) score for predicting the perioperative mortality of patients with cirrhosis. All studies supporting the use of these scoring systems, however, are retrospective and have not been prospectively validated.

The CTP classification is calculated using INR, albumin, bilirubin, and the presence or absence of encephalopathy and/or ascites;

TABLE 16.1 MORTALITY IN PATIENTS WITH CIRRHOSIS UNDERGOING ABDOMINAL SURGERY [1, 2, 4, 5]

Class A	5–6 points	~10 % mortality
Class B	7–9 points	~17–30 % mortality
Class C	10–15 points	~63–82 % mortality

calculators are widely available in textbooks and online. Table 16.1 shows approximate postoperative risk for CTP class A, B, and C.

Higher MELD scores generally correlate with worse outcomes [6–10]. For patients with MELD >15, the finding of serum albumin <2.5 has been shown to correlate with worse outcomes [11]. Calculators are widely available online to determine the MELD score. $MELD = 3.78 \times \log e$ (bilirubin in mg/dl) $+ 11.2 \times \log e$ (INR) $+ 9.57 \times \log e$ (creatinine in mg/dl) $+ 6.43$. Enter 1 for creatinine <1.0 or 4 for creatinine >4 or dialysis. Round to nearest integer. Mortality stratified by MELD score is shown in Table 16.2 [9].

The Mayo model (calculator available online) adds ASA classification to MELD score for the prediction of postoperative mortality [10]. It is based on a retrospective study of 772 patients with a median MELD of only 8, however, has not been prospectively validated, and should be applied to diverse populations with caution.

Figure 16.1 shows a risk stratification strategy for both acute hepatitis and chronic liver disease.

PERIOPERATIVE MANAGEMENT

PREOPERATIVE CONSIDERATIONS

Although the internist should refrain from making recommendations about intraoperative care, it is helpful to have some familiarity with issues that may arise during or as a result of anesthesia; these are well detailed elsewhere [12]. Consider making the following recommendations for patients proceeding to surgery:

- Delay surgery until after liver transplantation and/or suggest a less invasive option: cholecystostomy in place of cholecystectomy [13], etc.
- Preoperative TIPS may reduce perioperative GI bleeding for patients with severe portal hypertension, but at the expense of worsened encephalopathy [14, 15].

TABLE 16.2 POSTOPERATIVE MORTALITY OF PATIENTS WITH CIRRHOSIS AS PREDICTED BY MELD SCORE

MELD		5	10	15	20	25	30	35	40	45
Probability of death (%) (95 % CI)	All surgeries	5	7	11	17	26	36	50	59	67
		(2–13)	(3–15)	(6–19)	(11–25)	(17–38)	(21–53)	(27–73)	(31–82)	(34–89)
	Intra-abdominal surgeries	5	8	14	25	35	58	75	83	
		(1–16)	(3–20)	(7–27)	(15–39)	(21–51)	(34–79)	(43–92)	(48–96)	

Reprinted with permission from [9]

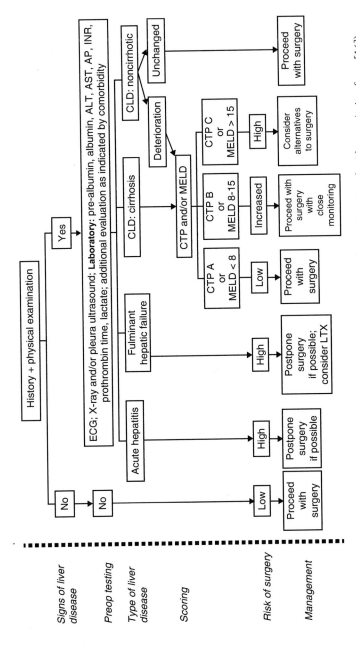

Fig. 16.1 Preoperative evaluation and risk stratification in suspected liver disease (reprinted with permission from [16])

- Treat ascites with diuretics (if peripheral edema is present), salt restriction, and/or paracentesis.
- Evaluate renal function preoperatively, recalling that calculated creatinine clearance may underestimate the degree of impairment.
- Correct coagulopathy with vitamin K and FFP and/or factor VIIA to normalize PT, plus or minus cryoprecipitate or DDAVP. FFP or factor VIIA, if given, should be given immediately before or during surgery due to short factor half-life and risk for volume overload.
- Keep extra cross-matched blood on hand, but note that transfusion may be associated with worsened outcomes [10].
- Consider transfusing platelets if severe thrombocytopenia is present; optimal goal of platelet count is unknown.

POSTOPERATIVE MANAGEMENT
- Watch clinically (consider ICU) for exacerbation of liver disease postoperatively: ascites, jaundice, encephalopathy, etc.
- Monitor renal function (BUN, Cr, electrolytes) and hepatic synthetic function (albumin, PT/INR, glucose) closely.
- Particularly after intra-abdominal surgery, patients experience significant third spacing and are susceptible to acute kidney injury: limit routine maintenance IV fluids postoperatively (to avoid exacerbating ascites and/or edema), but do not neglect to resuscitate an intravascularly volume-depleted patient.
- Be cautious with the use of diuretics for treatment of ascites or edema that may develop during the first couple of days after surgery while patients are still actively third-spacing fluids.
- Manage encephalopathy in the usual fashion (lactulose, rifaximin, etc.), and consider potential causes such as gastrointestinal bleeding, infection, medications, and the surgery itself.
- Use short-acting analgesics, such as fentanyl. Avoid benzodiazepines; if one must be used (i.e., to treat alcohol withdrawal), lorazepam is preferred.
- Avoid hypercarbia, which may cause splanchnic vasodilation and decrease portal blood flow.
- Use nonselective beta-blockade (unless contraindicated) and avoid fluid overload in patients with gastroesophageal varices.
- Optimize perioperative nutritional support.
- Limit acetaminophen use to not more than 2 g/day.

REFERENCES

1. Friedman LS. Surgery in the patient with liver disease. Trans Am Clin Climatol Assoc. 2010;121:102–204.
2. O'Leary JG. Surgery in the patient with liver disease. Clin Liver Dis. 2009;13(2):211–31.
3. Ribeireiro T, Swain J, et al. NAFLD and insulin resistance do not increase the risk of postoperative complications among patients undergoing bariatric surgery—a prospective analysis. Obes Surg. 2011;21(3):310–5.
4. Mansour A, Watson W, Shayani V, et al. Abdominal operations in patients with cirrhosis: still a major surgical challenge. Surgery. 1997;122(4):730–6.
5. Neeff H, Mariaskin D, Spangenberg HC, et al. Perioperative mortality after non-hepatic general surgery in patients with liver cirrhosis: an analysis of 138 operations in the 2000s using child and MELD scores. J Gastrointest Surg. 2011;15:1–11.
6. Farnsworth N, Fagan SP, Berger DH, et al. Child-Turcotte-Pugh versus MELD score as a predictor of outcome after elective and emergent surgery in cirrhotic patients. Am J Surg. 2004;188:580–3.
7. Perkins L, Jeffries M, Patel T. Utility of preoperative scores for predicting morbidity after cholecystectomy in patients with cirrhosis. Clin Gastroenterol Hepatol. 2004;2(12):1123–8.
8. Befeler AS, Palmer DE, Hoffman M, et al. The safety of intra-abdominal surgery in patients with cirrhosis: model for end-stage liver disease score is superior to Child-Turcotte-Pugh classification in predicting outcome. Arch Surg. 2005;140:650–4.
9. Northup PG, Wanamaker RC, Lee VD, et al. Model for end-stage liver disease (MELD) predicts nontransplant surgical mortality in patients with cirrhosis. Ann Surg. 2005;242(2):244–51.
10. Teh SH, Nagorney DM, Stevens SR, et al. Risk factors for mortality after surgery in patients with cirrhosis. Gastroenterology. 2007;132:1261–9.
11. Telem DA, Schiano T, Goldstone R, Han DK, Buch KE, Chin EH, Nguyen SQ, Divino CM. Factors that predict outcome of abdominal operations in patients with advanced cirrhosis. Clin Gastroenterol Hepatol. 2010;8:451–7.
12. Kiamanesh D, Rumley J, Moitra VK. Monitoring and managing hepatic disease in anaesthesia. Br J Anaesth. 2013;111 Suppl 1:i50–61.
13. Curro G, Lapichino G, Melita G, et al. Laparoscopic cholecystectomy in Child-Pugh class C cirrhotic patients. JSLS. 2005;9:311–5.
14. Azoulay D, Buabse F, Damiano I, et al. Neoadjuvant transjugular intrahepatic portosystemic shunt: a solution for extrahepatic abdominal operation in cirrhotic patients with severe portal hypertension. J Am Coll Surg. 2001;193(1):46–51.
15. Kim JJ, Narasimham LD, Yu E, Fontana RJ. Cirrhotic patients with a transjugular intrahepatic portosystemic shunt undergoing major extrahepatic surgery. J Clin Gastroenterol. 2009;43(6):574–9.
16. Hoetzel A, Ryan H, Schmidt R. Anesthetic considerations for the patient with liver disease. Curr Opin Anaesthesiol. 2012;25(3):340–7.

Chapter 17
Inflammatory Bowel Disease

Gabrielle Berger

BACKGROUND

Despite the widespread use of medical therapy in the management of inflammatory bowel disease (IBD), up to 30 % of patients with ulcerative colitis (UC) and 70 % of patients with Crohn's disease (CD) will require intra-abdominal surgery [1, 2]. Patients with IBD are at risk for postoperative complications including surgical site infection, intra-abdominal abscess, bacteremia, strictures and fistulae, small bowel obstruction, portal vein thrombosis, and poor wound healing including anastomotic leak and wound dehiscence [3–6].

This chapter focuses on evidence for IBD patients undergoing intra-abdominal surgery; however, the medication recommendations are applicable for IBD patients undergoing other types of surgery.

PREOPERATIVE EVALUATION

HISTORY AND PHYSICAL EXAMINATION
In addition to a standard comprehensive physical examination, the medical consultant should assess the patient for risk factors for post-surgical complications.

- Examine for fistulizing disease and evidence of intra-abdominal abscess
- Evaluate for symptoms of occult infection including fevers, chills, and night sweats
- Evaluate for symptoms of hypothalamic pituitary adrenal (HPA) axis suppression if glucocorticoids have been taken in the previous 3 months; observe for Cushingoid features (see Chap. 14)
- Assess for evidence of malnutrition

M.B. Jackson et al. (eds.), *The Perioperative Medicine Consult Handbook*, DOI 10.1007/978-3-319-09366-6_17, © Springer International Publishing Switzerland 2015

LABORATORY WORK-UP

- CBC—many immunomodulators used to treat IBD can cause anemia and leukopenia.
- Basic metabolic profile (BMP)—look for evidence of acute kidney injury (AKI) or chronic kidney disease (CKD) which can be caused by aminosalicylates and methotrexate.
- Consider liver function tests (LFTs)—some immunomodulators can cause hepatotoxicity.
- Glucose—need to optimize perioperative glycemic control if on glucocorticoids.

RISK STRATIFICATION

Most procedures for IBD are considered moderate or major surgeries and may involve a two- or three-stage operation. Several factors may increase the risk of morbidity and mortality.

- Patients with more extensive small bowel and colon involvement are at higher risk than those with only ileal involvement [7].
- Comorbid conditions such as malnutrition and anemia, as well as older age, may contribute to worse postoperative outcomes [5, 8].
- The use of glucocorticoids and narcotics has been associated with increased mortality and postoperative morbidity [7].

PERIOPERATIVE MANAGEMENT

MEDICATION MANAGEMENT

Appropriate perioperative medication management for patients with IBD remains challenging. Since the advent of biologic agents to control IBD (infliximab, adalimumab, and certolizumab pegol), numerous studies evaluating the postoperative complications in patients on anti-TNF alpha therapy have shown conflicting results. Most of these studies have been limited by retrospective design, small sample size, and an inability to control for confounders [9, 10]. However, current data and expert opinion indicate that anti-TNF alpha agents should be continued during the perioperative period [1, 2, 4, 6, 11, 12]. Additionally, many clinicians feel that patients on intermediate- and high-dose steroids should receive stress-dose steroids perioperatively (see Table 14.2 for dosing recommendations depending on preoperative dose and surgical risk) [8]. See Table 17.1 for other medication recommendations.

TABLE 17.1 MEDICATION MANAGEMENT DURING THE PERIOPERATIVE PERIOD[a]

Drug	Recommendation for practice	Evidence level[b]
Glucocorticoids	Continue; administer stress dose	
5-ASA	Discontinue on day of surgery and resume 3 days after surgery if normal renal function	C
Azathioprine, 6-MP	Discontinue on day of surgery and resume 3 days after surgery if normal renal function	B, C
Methotrexate	Continue, unless previous poor wound healing or postoperative infections	B, C
Cyclosporine	Continue but carefully monitor for opportunistic infectious complications	B, C
Infliximab	Continue without interruption	B

Adapted with permission from [8]
[a]5-ASA = 5-aminosalicylic acid; 6-MP = 6-mercaptopurine
[b]Evidence level A = multiple populations evaluated (trials and clinical registries), multiple randomized clinical trials, or meta-analysis; evidence level B = limited populations evaluated, data derived from a single randomized trial or nonrandomized studies; evidence level C = very limited populations evaluated or consensus opinion of experts, case studies, or standards of care

MONITORING/PREVENTION OF COMPLICATIONS

Patients undergoing surgery for IBD present clinicians with unique postoperative challenges that can delay recovery including limited options for pain management, hyperglycemia in patients on glucocorticoids, and poor nutritional status. The following measures may help guide clinicians in the appropriate postoperative management of these patients.

- Close attention to perioperative glycemic control for patients on glucocorticoids given that persistent hyperglycemia can delay wound healing and lead to surgical site complications.
- Attempt to minimize the use of narcotic analgesia, though it is important to note that narcotic agents are preferred over other pain medications, as studies have shown a possible association between NSAID use and IBD flares [13].
- Transfuse to maintain hemoglobin >7 g/dL.
- Close collaboration with nutrition colleagues to maintain adequate supplementation and aid postoperative healing—patients

may need TPN depending on underlying malnutrition and disease severity particularly if patient is undergoing a two- or three-stage procedure.

■ Early antibiotic therapy and surgical exploration if concerned for intra-abdominal source of sepsis.

REFERENCES

1. Narula N, Charleton D, Marshall JK. Meta-analysis: peri-operative anti-TNFα treatment and post-operative complications in patients with inflammatory bowel disease. Aliment Pharmacol Ther. 2013;37(11):1057–64. doi:10.1111/apt.12313.
2. Nasir BS, Dozois EJ, Cima RR, et al. Perioperative anti-tumor necrosis factor therapy does not increase the rate of early postoperative complications in Crohn's disease. J Gastrointest Surg. 2010;14(12):1859–66. doi:10.1007/s11605-010-1341-5.
3. Appau KA, Fazio VW, Shen B, et al. Use of infliximab within 3 months of ileocolonic resection is associated with adverse postoperative outcomes in Crohn's patients. J Gastrointest Surg. 2008;12(10):1738–44. doi:10.1007/s11605-008-0646-0.
4. Bafford AC, Powers S, Ha C, et al. Immunosuppressive therapy does not increase operative morbidity in patients with Crohn's disease. J Clin Gastroenterol. 2013;47(6):491–5. doi:10.1097/MCG.0b013e3182677003.
5. Beddy D, Dozois EJ, Pemberton JH. Perioperative complications in inflammatory bowel disease. Inflamm Bowel Dis. 2011;17(7):1610–9. doi:10.1002/ibd.21504.
6. Kunitake H, Hodin R, Shellito PC, Sands BE, Korzenik J, Bordeianou L. Perioperative treatment with infliximab in patients with Crohn's disease and ulcerative colitis is not associated with an increased rate of postoperative complications. J Gastrointest Surg. 2008;12(10):1730–7. doi:10.1007/s11605-008-0630-8.
7. Lichtenstein GR, Feagan BG, Cohen RD, et al. Serious infection and mortality in patients with Crohn's disease: more than 5 years of follow-up in the TREAT™ registry. Am J Gastroenterol. 2012;107(9):1409–22. doi:10.1038/ajg.2012.218.
8. Kumar A, Auron M, Aneja A, Mohr F, Jain A, Shen B. Inflammatory bowel disease: perioperative pharmacological considerations. Mayo Clin Proc. 2011;86(8):748–57. doi:10.4065/mcp.2011.0074.
9. Sewell JL, Mahadevan U. Infliximab and surgical complications: truth or perception? Gastroenterology. 2009;136(1):354–5. doi:10.1053/j.gastro.2008.11.057.
10. Ali T. Risk of post-operative complications associated with anti-TNF therapy in inflammatory bowel disease. WJG. 2012;18(3):197. doi:10.3748/wjg.v18.i3.197.
11. Nørgård BM, Nielsen J, Qvist N, Gradel KO, de Muckadell OBS, Kjeldsen J. Pre-operative use of anti-TNF-α agents and the risk of post-operative complications in patients with Crohn's disease – a nationwide cohort study. Aliment Pharmacol Ther. 2012;37(2):214–24. doi:10.1111/apt.12159.
12. Nørgård BM, Nielsen J, Qvist N, Gradel KO, Muckadell OBS, Kjeldsen J. Pre-operative use of anti-TNF-α agents and the risk of post-operative complications in patients with ulcerative colitis – a nationwide cohort study. Aliment Pharmacol Ther. 2012;35(11):1301–9. doi:10.1111/j.1365-2036.2012.05099.x.
13. Singh S, Graff LA, Bernstein CN. Do NSAIDs, antibiotics, infections, or stress trigger flares in IBD? Am J Gastroenterol. 2009;104(5):1298–314. doi:10.1038/ajg.2009.15.

Chapter 18
Chronic Anticoagulation

Kelly Wentworth and Sabeena Setia

BACKGROUND

Patients receiving chronic anticoagulation often require interruption of treatment perioperatively. It remains challenging to mitigate both the risk of thromboembolic events off anticoagulation and the risk of surgical bleeding on anticoagulation. The underlying condition requiring anticoagulation impacts the decision of whether to interrupt long-acting agents such as warfarin or to use bridging therapy with shorter-acting agents. For further discussion of perioperative management of patients receiving anticoagulation for atrial fibrillation and venous thromboembolic disease, please refer to Chaps. 9 and 31.

PREOPERATIVE EVALUATION

When assessing a patient who is chronically anticoagulated, it is important to consider and document the following:

- Specific indication for anticoagulation
- Anticoagulant in use and any recent dose adjustments
- Evaluation of medications which may interact with the anticoagulant
- History of bleeding complications
- Whether bridging was recommended in the past
- Plan developed with the patient's anticoagulation clinic
- Coagulation panel and complete blood count
- Potential need for nerve/neuraxial catheter for anesthesia/analgesia perioperatively

M.B. Jackson et al. (eds.), *The Perioperative Medicine Consult Handbook*, DOI 10.1007/978-3-319-09366-6_18,
© Springer International Publishing Switzerland 2015

PERIOPERATIVE MANAGEMENT

RISK STRATIFICATION FOR BRIDGING PATIENTS WHO ARE CHRONICALLY ANTICOAGULATED

In general, patients who are high risk for thrombus formation should be bridged, and those who are low risk should not be bridged. For patients at intermediate risk of thrombus formation, the decision to bridge should be based on surgery-related factors and the individual patient's condition (see Fig. 18.1).

Many minor procedures may be performed while on therapeutic anticoagulation due to lower bleeding risk and the ability for local control measures to obtain hemostasis (see Table 18.1). One should always discuss this with the surgeon. An INR should be checked to ensure that the patient's anticoagulation is not supratherapeutic.

Risk Stratum and Recommendations for Use of Bridge Therapy	Indication for Warfarin Therapy			
	Mechanical Heart Valve	Atrial Fibrillation	Venous Thromboembolism	Low Ejection Fraction with Normal Sinus Rhythm
	from Peri-operative management of antithrombotic therapy: Antithrombotic Therapy and Prevention of Thrombosis, 9th Edition. American College of Chest Physicians Evidence Based Clinical Practice Guidelines. Chest 2012; 141 (suppl 2): e326s – e350s.			*from* UWMedicine Division of Cardiology
HIGH RISK *Recommendation:* **Use bridging (Grade 2C)**	• any mitral valve prosthesis • older (caged-ball or tilting disc) aortic valve prosthesis • recent (within 6 months) stroke or transient ischemic attack	• CHADS₂ score of 5 or 6 • recent (within 3 months) stroke or transient ischemic attack • rheumatic valvular heart disease	• recent (within 3 months) VTE • severe thrombophilia (e.g., deficiency of protein C, protein S or antithrombin, antiphospholipid antibodies, or multiple abnormalities)	• mural thrombus present on echo • documented mural thrombus in the past 3 months • history of cardioembolic stroke
RISK MODERATE *Recommendation:* **Determine bridging vs not bridging based on assessment of individual patient and surgery-related factors (Not Graded)**	• bileaflet aortic valve prosthesis and one of the following: atrial fibrillation, prior stroke or transient ischemic attack, hypertension, diabetes, congestive heart failure, age >75 years	• CHADS₂ score of 3 of 4	• VTE within the past 3 to 12 months *(consider VTE prophylaxis rather than full intensity bridge therapy)* • non-severe thrombophilic conditions (e.g., heterozygous factor V Leiden mutation heterozygous factor II mutation) • recurrent VTE • active cancer (treated within 6 months or palliative)	• history of mural thrombus with persistent risk factors (apical akinesis, LV aneurysm, dilated LV)
LOW RISK *Recommendation:* **Do not use bridging (Grade 2C)**	• bileaflet aortic valve prosthesis without atrial fibrillation and no other risk factors for stroke	• CHADS₂ score of 0 to 2 (no prior stroke or transient ischemic attack)	• single VTE occurred greater than 12 months ago and no other risk factors	• no history of mural thrombus

Fig. 18.1 University of Washington risk stratum and recommendations for use of bridge therapy [1, 2] (Reprinted with permission from [3])

TABLE 18.1 ANTICOAGULATION MANAGEMENT FOR MINOR PROCEDURES [2]

Cataract surgery	Stopping warfarin is usually not indicated
Other ophthalmologic procedures	Should be decided on a case-by-case basis
Dermatology	Stopping warfarin is usually not indicated unless the surgery is extensive
Dental surgery	Stopping warfarin is usually not indicated except in very large cases or bone excision Consider adding an oral pro-hemostatic agent such as aminocaproic acid mouthwash postoperatively

Reprinted with permission from [3]

STRATEGIES FOR REVERSAL OF COMMON ANTICOAGULANTS

Consider whether the indication is for active bleeding or reversal for surgery and the time period over which you wish to reverse anticoagulation. See Fig. 18.2 for specific recommendations. Important points include the following:

- IV vitamin K: Acts quickly and reverses quickly. Useful if you seek to reverse warfarin effect within 24 h. There is a risk of anaphylaxis with the IV form.
- Oral vitamin K: There is reasonable data showing that low-dose oral vitamin K may be used to reverse warfarin effect with similar efficacy as IV vitamin K (note different dosing) at 24 h, although IV administration acts more quickly in the first few hours [4]. Be careful not to overdose oral vitamin K if reversing with the intention of reestablishing therapeutic anticoagulation with warfarin in the near future.
- SC vitamin K: The data for SC vitamin K is sufficiently mixed such that oral or IV is preferred.
- Avoid vitamin K administration in patients with a mechanical valve who will be undergoing surgery as this may induce a hypercoagulable state.
- Fresh frozen plasma (FFP): Acts quickly, but also is effective for a relatively short duration. Useful immediately prior to procedure (e.g., less than 12 h) or for any indication where rapid reversal is required; it may have to be re-dosed or vitamin K concurrently administered if prolonged reversal of anticoagulation is required.

GENERIC (BRAND) NAMES	ELIMINATION HALF-LIFE	REMOVED BY HD	STRATEGIES TO REVERSE OR MINIMIZE DRUG EFFECT	
apixaban (Eliquis)	8-15 hours (longer in renal impairment)	NO	• Drug activity can be assessed with anti-factor Xa activity assay (UWMedicine: use Heparin Activity for LMWH [LMWXa]: not calibrated for apixaban) • If ingested within 2 hours, administer activated charcoal • Consider 4-factor PCC (KCentra) 50 units/kg (maximum 5000 units) NOTE: PCC may partially correct PT/aPTT but will not affect anti-factor Xa activity and will not increase drug clearance; correlation of shortening PT/aPTT with reduction in bleeding risk is unknown	
argatroban	40-50 minutes	~20%	• Turn off infusion • Degree of reversal can be assessed with PTT and/or plasma-diluted thrombin time (UWMedicine: DTI assay [DTIPAT])	
bivalirudin (Aggrastat)	25 minutes (up to 1 hr in severe renal impairment)	~25%	• Turn off infusion • Degree of reversal can be assessed with plasma-diluted thrombin time (UWMedicine: DTI assay [DTIPAT])	
dabigatran (Pradaxa)	14-17 hours (up to 34 hrs in severe renal impairment)	~65%	• Drug activity can be assessed with aPTT and/or plasma-diluted thrombin time (UWMedicine: dabigatran assay [DABIG]) • If ingested within 2 hours, administer activated charcoal • Consider 4-factor PCC (KCentra) 50 units/kg (maximum 5000 units) NOTE: PCC may partially correct aPTT and plasma-diluted thrombin time but will not increase drug clearance; correlation of lab results with reduction in bleeding risk is unknown	

| dalteparin (Fragmin) enoxaparin (Lovenox) | 3-5 hours (longer in renal impairment) | ~20% | • Use protamine for partial neutralization (~60%)
 • Degree of reversal can be assessed with anti factor Xa activity (UWMedicine: anti-Xa for LMWH [LMWXA]) | |

Time since last dose of LMWH	Dose of protamine for each 100 units of dalteparin or 1mg of enoxaparin administered	
< 8 hrs	1mg	(or 50mg fixed dose)
8-12 hrs	0.5mg	(or 25mg fixed dose)
> 12 hrs	Not likely to be useful	(or 25mg fixed dose)

| fondaparinux (Arixtra) | 17–21 hours (significantly longer in renal impairment) | NO | • Fondaparinux levels can be assessed by anti-factor Xa activity (UWMedicine: fondaparinux assay [FNDXT])
 • Consider rFVIIa (Novoseven) 90 mcg/kg
 NOTE: rVIIa will not effect anti-factor Xa activity and will not increase drug clearance | |
| Heparin | 30–90 minutes (dose dependent) | Partial | • Use protamine for heparin neutralization (100%)
 • Degree of reversal can be assessed with PTT and/or anti factor Xa activity (UWMedicine: Heparin Activity for Heparin [HIXA] | |

Time since last dose of heparin	Dose of protamine for each 100 units of heparin administered	
Immediate	1mg	(or 25mg fixed dose)
30 minutes – 2 hrs	0.5mg	(or 10mg fixed dose)
>2 hrs	0.25mg	(or 10mg fixed dose)

| Rivaroxaban (Xarelto) | Healthy: 5-9 hrs
 Elderly: 11-13 hrs
 (longer in renal impairment) | NO | • Drug activity can be assessed with anti-factor Xa activity (UWMedicine: rivaroxaban assay [RIVA])
 • If ingested within 2 hours, administer activated charcoal
 • Consider 4-factor PCC (KCentra) 50 units/kg (maximum 5000 units)
 NOTE: PCC may partially correct PT/aPTT but will not affect anti-factor Xa activity and will not increase drug clearance; correlation of shortening PT/aPTT with reduction in bleeding risk is unknown | |

Fig. 18.2 University of Washington strategies to reverse or minimize drug effect of common anticoagulants (Reprinted with permission from [3])

Warfarin (Coumadin)	INR	CLINICAL SCENARIO	MANAGEMENT
	<4.5	No bleeding	• Hold warfarin until INR in therapeutic range
		Rapid reversal required	• Hold warfarin • Consider vitamin K 2.5mg oral
	4.5-10	No bleeding	• Hold warfarin until INR in therapeutic range • Consider vitamin K 2.5mg oral
		Rapid reversal required	• Hold warfarin • Give vitamin K 2.5mg oral or 1mg IV infusion *(IV administration of vitamin K has faster onset of action)*
	>10	No bleeding	• Hold warfarin until INR in therapeutic range • Give vitamin K 2.5mg oral or 1-2mg IV infusion over 30 minutes, and repeat q24h as needed *(IV administration of vitamin K has faster onset of action)*
		Rapid reversal required	• Hold warfarin • Give vitamin K 1-2mg IV infusion over 30 minutes, and repeat q6-24h as needed

	Any INR	Serious or life-threatening bleeding	• Hold warfarin
			• Give vitamin K 10mg IV infusion over 30 minutes
			• Give 4 units FFP/plasma
			• OR consider 4-factor PCC (Kcentra)
			  (preferred for life-threatening bleeding)
			
			  INR 1.5 – 3.9: 25 units/kg (maximum 2500 units)
			  INR 4.0 – 6.0: 35 units/kg (maximum 3500 units)
			  INR > 6.0: 50 units/kg (maximum 5000 units)

Fig. 18.2 (continued)

ANTICOAGULATION IN PATIENTS WITH NEURAXIAL CATHETERS

If patients receiving chronic anticoagulation require neuraxial catheters for analgesia/anesthesia during the perioperative period, please note that therapeutic-dose anticoagulation is contraindicated while the catheter is in place, although there are exceptions. Figure 18.3 summarizes recommendations from the University of Washington Medical Center.

MEDICATION	PRIOR TO NEURAXIAL/NERVE PROCEDURE	WHILE NEURAXIAL/NERVE CATHETER IN PLACE	AFTER NEURAXIAL/NERVE PROCEDURE
	Minimum time between last dose of anticoagulant and spinal injection OR neuraxial/ nerve catheter placement	Restrictions on use of anticoagulants while neuraxial/nerve catheters are in place and prior to their removal	Minimum time between neuraxial/nerve catheter removal OR spinal/nerve injection and next anticoagulant dose
ANTICOAGULANTS FOR VTE PROPHYLAXIS			
heparin unfractionated 5000 units q8 or q12 hr	May be given; no time restrictions for catheter placement/removal or spinal injections Do NOT call Pain Service		
heparin unfractionated 7500 units SQ q8 hr	8 hrs	CONTRAINDICATED while catheter in place: may NOT be given unless approved by Pain Service Attending	4 hrs
dalteparin (Fragmin) 5000 units SQ qday	12 hrs (longer in renal impairment)	May be given BUT: •Must wait 8 hrs after catheter PLACEMENT before giving dose •Must wait 12 hrs after last dose before REMOVING catheter	4 hrs
enoxaparin (Lovenox) 40mg SQ qday			
enoxaparin (Lovenox) 30mg SQ q12 hr or 40mg SQ q12 hr	12 hrs (longer in renal impairment)	CONTRAINDICATED while catheter in place: may NOT be given unless approved by Pain Service Attending	4 hrs
fondaparinux (Arixtra) < 2.5mg SQ qday	48 hrs (longer in renal impairment)		
rivaroxaban (Xarelto) 10mg po qday	24 hrs (longer in renal impairment)	May be given BUT contact Pain Service regarding dose timing •Must wait 8 hrs after catheter PLACEMENT before giving dose •Must wait 12 hrs after last dose before REMOVING catheter	6 hrs (per manufacturer recommendations)
AGENTS USED FOR FULL SYSTEMIC ANTICOAGULATION			
dabigatran (Pradaxa)	72 hrs (longer in renal impairment)	CONTRAINDICATED while catheter in place: may NOT be given unless approved by Pain Service Attending	4 hrs
dalteparin (Fragmin) 200 Units/kg SQ qday or 100 Units/kg SQ q12 hr	24 hrs (longer in renal impairment)		
enoxaparin (Lovenox) 1.5mg/kg SQ qday or 1mg/kg SQ q12 hr	24 hrs (longer in renal impairment)		
fondaparinux (Arixtra) 5-10mg SQ qday	72 hrs (longer in renal impairment)		
heparin unfractionated IV continuous infusion or >5000 Units SQ bid or tid	when aPTT<40 sec		
rivaroxaban (Xarelto) 15-20mg po qday	24 hrs (longer in renal impairment)		6 hrs (per manufacturer recommendations)
warfarin (Coumadin)	when INR< 1.5		4 hrs

ATTENTION! WHEN CAN YOU SAFELY DO NEURAXIAL/PERIPHERAL NERVE PROCEDURES OR GIVE ANTICOAGULANTS?
Neuraxial routes include epidural and intrathecal infusions, implanted intrathecal pumps, and spinal injections. Peripheral routes include all peripheral nerve and plexus infusions. NOTE: Bloody tap/procedure? Anesthesia to call Pain Service

Fig. 18.3 University of Washington recommendations for anticoagulant management in the setting of neuraxial catheters (Reprinted with permission from [3])

REFERENCES

1. Bonow RO, Carabellow BA, Chatterjee K, et al. 2008 Focused update incorporated into the ACC/AHA 2006 guidelines for the management of patients with valvular heart disease. J Am Coll Cardiol. 2008;52:e1–142.
2. Douketis JD, Spyropoulos AC, Spencer FA, et al. Perioperative management of antithrombotic therapy: antithrombotic therapy and prevention of thrombosis, 9th ed: American College of Chest Physicians Evidence-Based Clinical Practice Guidelines. Chest. 2012;141:e326S–50.
3. UWMC Anticoagulation Clinic website. http://depts.washington.edu/anticoag. Accessed October 2014.
4. Lubetsky A, Yonath H, Olchovsky D, et al. Comparison of oral vs intravenous phytonadione (vitamin K1) in patients with excessive anticoagulation: a prospective randomized controlled study. Arch Intern Med. 2003;163:2469–74.

Chapter 19
Disorders of Hemostasis

Ronald Huang

BACKGROUND

Assessing the risk of perioperative bleeding is a fundamental component of the preoperative evaluation. Early recognition and proper perioperative management of hemostatic disorders is important to prevent and reduce unexpected and unnecessary bleeding.

PREOPERATIVE EVALUATION

ESTIMATION OF PROCEDURAL BLEEDING RISK
- The risk of perioperative bleeding depends upon both the presence or absence of normal hemostasis and the type of procedure being performed.
- Procedures can be classified as having a low, moderate, or high risk of bleeding based on whether vital organs are involved, the amount of surgical dissection, exposure of the surgical site, likelihood of a complication adversely affecting the outcome of surgery, and frequency of bleeding complications (see Table 19.1).

HISTORY AND PHYSICAL
A *hemostatic history* should be obtained on all patients regardless of the procedure being performed [1–4]. Patients should be asked about:
- Personal history of abnormal bleeding, blood transfusion, easy bruising, and excessive bleeding associated with child birth, menses, minor trauma, or surgery (including dental procedures or tonsillectomy)
- Family history of bleeding disorders
- Past medical history of hepatic, renal, or hematologic disease

M.B. Jackson et al. (eds.), *The Perioperative Medicine Consult Handbook*, DOI 10.1007/978-3-319-09366-6_19,
© Springer International Publishing Switzerland 2015

TABLE 19.1 RISK OF BLEEDING WITH SURGICAL OR INVASIVE PROCEDURES

Risk	Type of procedure	Examples
Low	Non-vital organs involved, exposed surgical site, limited dissection	Lymph node biopsy, dental extraction, cataract extraction, most cutaneous surgery, laparoscopic procedures, coronary angiography
Moderate	Vital organs involved, deep or extensive dissection	Laparotomy, thoracotomy, mastectomy, major orthopedic surgery, pacemaker insertion
High	Bleeding likely to compromise surgical result, bleeding complications frequent	Neurosurgery, ophthalmic surgery, cardiopulmonary bypass, prostatectomy, bladder surgery, major vascular surgery, renal biopsy, bowel polypectomy

Reprinted with permission from [3]

- Current medication use, including aspirin, over-the-counter pain medications, antiplatelet medications, or anticoagulants, and vitamins, supplements, or herbal preparations

Physical exam may:
- Suggest the presence of a hemostatic disorder (e.g. petechiae, purpura, ecchymoses)
- Demonstrate chronic findings of hemostatic disorders (e.g., joint deformity and muscle atrophy in hemophiliacs)
- Reveal signs of chronic conditions that result in hemostatic abnormalities (e.g., jaundice, ascites, and spider telangiectasias in cirrhosis, or pallor, lymphadenopathy, and splenomegaly in hematologic disease)

TESTING
Routine preoperative laboratory testing, including platelet count, prothrombin time (PT/INR), and partial thromboplastin time (PTT), is generally not indicated for patients without a positive bleeding history [5–11]. Testing should be performed as indicated by the history and the procedural bleeding risk:
- For low-risk procedures, if the history is reassuring for normal hemostasis, no further testing is required.
- For high-risk procedures, and to a lesser degree for moderate-risk procedures, a platelet count, PT/INR, and PTT may be considered in addition to history [3].

- For any procedure, initial testing for patients with a suspected disorder of hemostasis should include a platelet count, PT/INR, and PTT.

PERIOPERATIVE MANAGEMENT

THROMBOCYTOPENIA

- Thrombocytopenia (platelet count <150,000/µL) may be due to decreased production (e.g. medications, chemotherapy, hematologic disease, viral infection), splenic sequestration (e.g. liver disease), or increased destruction (e.g. immune thrombocytopenia, systemic lupus erythematosus).
- Platelet counts may also be falsely low due to platelet clumping caused by EDTA in blood collection tubes (pseudothrombocytopenia).
- Postoperative thrombocytopenia and heparin-induced thrombocytopenia (HIT) are discussed in Chaps. 20 and 21.
- Unexplained thrombocytopenia should be evaluated prior to elective surgery. The initial evaluation should include a complete history and physical examination, a repeat CBC, and a peripheral blood smear. Additional testing will depend on the history and physical examination.
- Both elective and emergent surgical procedures can be safely performed for most patients with thrombocytopenia or platelet dysfunction with the use of platelet transfusions. Recommendations for platelet transfusion for the surgical patient are listed in Table 19.2.

Effect of Platelet Transfusions

- Platelet transfusions are either pooled (random donor) platelets or apheresis (single donor) platelets.
- A unit of pooled platelets (50–60 mL) is prepared from platelets that have been separated from a unit of whole blood. Five or six units of pooled platelets from separate donors are usually combined into a single bag for transfusion, called a "five-" or "six-pack."
- A unit of apheresis platelets (150–300 mL) is collected from a single donor.
- The effect of platelet transfusions is variable, but 4–6 units of pooled platelets or a single unit of apheresis platelets is expected to increase the platelet count by 30–60,000/µL in an average-sized patient.

TABLE 19.2 RECOMMENDATIONS FOR PLATELET TRANSFUSION FOR THE SURGICAL PATIENT [10, 11]

Plts <50,000/μL—platelet transfusion is indicated for the surgical patient

Plts 50,000–100,000/μL—considered adequate for most procedures, except for central nervous system (CNS) procedures for which platelet transfusion is indicated for platelet count <100,000/μL

Plts >100,000/μL—platelet transfusion is usually not necessary, but may be indicated if there is known or suspected platelet dysfunction or there is ongoing or anticipated bleeding

- A posttransfusion platelet count can be sent 10–60 min after transfusion to assess for response. The platelet count will gradually fall to pre-transfusion levels after 2–3 days.
- If a patient does not respond to platelet transfusions, a pre- and posttransfusion platelet count should be obtained.
- A patient is refractory to platelet transfusions if the platelet count fails to increase by 10,000/μL. The next step is to send panel reactive antibody (PRA) to test for the presence of HLA antibodies. If the patient has a high or a positive PRA, apheresis platelets should be collected from an HLA-matched donor for transfusion.

IMMUNE THROMBOCYTOPENIA

- Immune thrombocytopenia (ITP) is characterized by platelet destruction from platelet autoantibodies.
- The prevalence of ITP in adults is estimated to be 9.5–23.6 per 100,000 persons [12].
- ITP often presents as asymptomatic thrombocytopenia, but patients may also present with bleeding (petechiae, mucocutaneous bleeding).
- ITP in adults has a gradual onset and follows a chronic or remitting and relapsing course.
- ITP is a diagnosis of exclusion. Nonimmune causes of thrombocytopenia (e.g., splenic sequestration, hematologic disease) and secondary causes of ITP (e.g., HIV, HCV, drug-induced, or autoimmune) should be considered prior to making a diagnosis of ITP. If ITP is suspected, a hematologist should be consulted for evaluation prior to surgery.
- For elective procedures, patients with ITP are treated preoperatively with intravenous immunoglobulin (IVIG) and/or steroids to increase the platelet count to adequate levels such that transfusion is not needed. Newer therapies for patients with chronic

ITP in nonsurgical settings include rituximab and thrombopoietin mimetics (romiplostim and eltrombopag), but their role in
the perioperative setting is not studied [12]. Consultation with
a hematologist is advised to guide perioperative management.
- When thrombocytopenia is due to increased platelet destruction (e.g., ITP), platelet transfusions are less effective and are
reserved for emergent procedures or life-threatening bleeding.
For patients with ITP, IVIG and steroids are also used for emergent procedures.

PLATELET DYSFUNCTION
- Platelet dysfunction is most commonly due to medications
(e.g., NSAIDs, aspirin, clopidogrel), but may also be due to
other conditions such as uremia. Inherited causes of platelet
dysfunction are rare.
- If history and physical suggests platelet disorder without a
readily apparent explanation and the platelet count is normal,
then a test of platelet function (e.g., platelet function analyzer
PFA-100) should be considered to screen for platelet dysfunction. Testing for von Willebrand disease should also be considered in these settings.
- Medications should be reviewed and managed accordingly
around the time of surgery (see Chap. 4).
- Platelet dysfunction due to uremia is managed with dialysis,
desmopressin, and raising hemoglobin to 10 g/dL.

VON WILLEBRAND DISEASE
- Von Willebrand disease (VWD) is the most common inherited
bleeding disorder. The prevalence of VWD has been estimated
to be as high as 1 % of the general population, but clinically
significant VWD is far less common [13, 14].
- Von Willebrand factor (VWF) mediates the adhesion of platelets
to damaged endothelium and binds and stabilizes factor VIII.
Von Willebrand disease (VWD) is caused by a deficiency or dysfunction of VWF, which may also result in low factor VIII levels.
- Type 1 and 3 VWD represent a mild or severe deficiency of
VWF, respectively; type 2 VWD represents a group of four
subtypes that are characterized by dysfunctional VWF.
- If a diagnosis of VWD is suspected, initial laboratory testing
should include VWF antigen, VWF activity (e.g., ristocetin
cofactor activity), and factor VIII activity levels. Referral to a
hematologist for more specialized testing and treatment is recommended if any studies are abnormal.

- Although routine prophylaxis is generally not required for patients with VWD, surgical prophylaxis with desmopressin, factor VIII/VWF concentrates, antifibrinolytic therapy, or some combination of the three is recommended, as is consultation with a hematologist, as the treatment may vary considerably depending on the VWD type.

- Desmopressin is most effective for type 1 VWD as it transiently increases VWF and factor VIII levels by 2–5 times [13, 14]. Prior to using desmopressin for surgical prophylaxis, patients should receive a test dose of desmopressin to establish responsiveness. For those patients who respond to desmopressin, the recommended dose of desmopressin is 0.3 µg/kg IV infused over 30 min. Desmopressin should be administered every 12–24 h if needed. Tachyphylaxis is common and response to desmopressin is generally diminished after 2–4 doses. Factor VIII activity and VWF activity should be monitored for continued response. Fluid intake should be limited during treatment with desmopressin use due to the rare risk of hyponatremia. Desmopressin should not be used in patients with unstable coronary artery disease.

- For those patients with VWD who are not candidates for desmopressin, factor VIII/VWF concentrates are recommended for surgical prophylaxis. Dosing is based on the type of surgery and generally ranges from 20 to 60 IU/kg every 8–24 h [13, 14]. For minor surgery, VWF activity and factor VIII activity levels should be maintained >30 IU/dL for 1–5 days. For major surgery, initial target VWF activity and factor VIII activity levels should be ≥100 IU/dL, then should be maintained at >50 IU/dL for 5–14 days after major surgery.

ACQUIRED DISORDERS OF COAGULATION

- Acquired disorders of coagulation from liver disease, vitamin K deficiency, and anticoagulants are common. Perioperative management of patients with liver disease and anticoagulants are discussed in Chaps. 16 and 18.

- Vitamin K deficiency should be suspected in patients with an elevated PT/INR that corrects with 1:1 mixing study and the appropriate clinical context (inadequate dietary intake or TPN, antibiotics, disease of malabsorption, liver disease).

- Patients with suspected vitamin K deficiency and coagulopathy are easily treated prior to surgery. For elective surgeries, oral vitamin K (5–10 mg daily) is recommended, and the PT/INR should be repeated prior to surgery. For more urgent or emergent surgeries, intravenous vitamin K (1–2.5 mg IV once) is usually sufficient, but correction with fresh frozen plasma (FFP) may be necessary.

Effect of Fresh Frozen Plasma Transfusions

- One unit of fresh frozen plasma (FFP) is the plasma collected from a unit of whole blood. The volume of one unit of FFP is roughly 200–300 mL.
- FFP contains all coagulation factors in normal or mildly reduced concentrations. The recommended dose of FFP is 10–15 mL/kg of body weight. Since one unit of FFP is ~250 mL, 2–4 units of FFP are necessary for a therapeutic effect. A posttransfusion PT/INR and/or PTT should be measured 15–30 min after transfusion to monitor for desired response.

INHERITED COAGULATION FACTOR DEFICIENCIES

- Inherited factor deficiencies are rare, especially when compared with acquired coagulopathies. The most common of the inherited factor deficiencies are hemophilia A (factor VIII deficiency) and hemophilia B (factor IX deficiency). The prevalence of hemophilia A is approximately 1:10,000 males, and the prevalence of hemophilia B is 1:50,000 males [15]. Female carriers of hemophilia A or B may have bleeding symptoms, although usually less severe than in males.
- There is some variability depending on the severity of the factor deficiency, but patients with hemophilia are usually diagnosed as children and are followed by a hematologist. Patients with hemophilia should receive recombinant factor or plasma-derived factor for surgical prophylaxis. Dosing will vary based on the severity of the hemophilia and the surgery being performed, but in general for major surgeries enough factor should initially be given to reach >100 % of factor VIII or factor IX activity [15]. Patients should continue to receive factor replacement to maintain factor levels >50 % for several days (e.g., 10–14 days for joint replacement) following surgery [15]. Factor activity levels should be monitored postoperatively. Consultation with a hematologist is recommended.

REFERENCES

1. Rapaport SI. Preoperative hemostatic evaluation: which tests, if any? Blood. 1983;61(2): 229–31.
2. Chee YL, Crawford JC, Watson HG, et al. Guidelines on the assessment of bleeding risk prior to surgery or invasive procedures. British Committee for Standards in Haematology. Br J Haematol. 2008;140(5):496–504.
3. Reding MT, Key NS. Hematologic problems in the surgical patient: bleeding and thrombosis. In: Hoffman R, Benz RJ, Shattil S, et al., editors. Hematology: basic principles and practice. 6th ed. Philadelphia, PA: Saunders; 2013. p. 2234.
4. Sramek A, Eikenboom JC, Briet E, et al. Usefulness of patient interview in bleeding disorders. Arch Intern Med. 1995;155(13):1409–15.
5. Kaplan EB, Sheiner LB, Boeckmann AJ, et al. The usefulness of preoperative laboratory screening. JAMA. 1985;253(24):3576–81.
6. Blery C, Charpak Y, Szatan M, et al. Evaluation of a protocol for selective ordering of preoperative tests. Lancet. 1986;1(8473):139–41.
7. Rohrer MJ, Michelotti MC, Nahrwold DL. A prospective evaluation of the efficacy of preoperative coagulation testing. Ann Surg. 1988;208(5):554–7.
8. Houry S, Georgeac C, Hay JM, et al. A prospective multicenter evaluation of preoperative hemostatic screening tests. The French Associations for Surgical Research. Am J Surg. 1995;170(1):19–23.
9. Eckman MH, Erban JK, Singh SK, et al. Screening for the risk for bleeding or thrombosis. Ann Intern Med. 2003;138(3):W15–24.
10. American Society of Anesthesiologists Task Force on Perioperative Blood Transfusion and Adjuvant Therapies. Practice guidelines for perioperative blood transfusion and adjuvant therapies: an updated report by the American Society of Anesthesiologists Task Force on Perioperative Blood Transfusion and Adjuvant Therapies. Anesthesiology. 2006;105(1): 198–208.
11. British Committee for Standards in Haematology, Blood Transfusion Task Force. Guidelines for the use of platelet transfusions. Br J Haematol. 2003;122(1):10–23.
12. Lakshmanan S, Cuker A. Contemporary management of primary immune thrombocytopenia in adults. J Thromb Haemost. 2012;10(10):1988–98.
13. Nichols WL, Hultin MB, James AH, et al. von Willebrand disease (VWD): evidence-based diagnosis and management guidelines, the National Heart, Lung, and Blood Institute (NHLBI) Expert Panel report (USA). Haemophilia. 2008;14(2):171–232.
14. Castaman G, Goodeve A, Eikenboom J, European Group on von Willebrand Disease. Principles of care for the diagnosis and treatment of von Willebrand disease. Haematologica. 2013;98(5):667–74.
15. Carcao M, Moorehead P, Lillicrap D. Hemophilia A and B. In: Hoffman R, Benz EJ, Silberstein LE, et al., editors. Hematology: basic principles and practice. 6th ed. Philadelphia, PA: Saunders; 2013. p. 1940.

Chapter 20
Thrombocytopenia

Elizabeth Kaplan

BACKGROUND

Thrombocytopenia, defined as a platelet count <150,000 [1], is a common hematologic abnormality after major surgery, although the actual incidence is not reported in the literature [2]. Generally, platelets >50,000 are not associated with significant bleeding. Spontaneous bleeding usually does not occur with platelets >20,000. Patients may have multiple possible causes of postoperative thrombocytopenia, some with grave consequences. It is important to distinguish between these etiologies for the individual patient and intervene early to prevent morbidity.

PERIOPERATIVE MANAGEMENT

ASSESSMENT
Postoperative thrombocytopenia can be due to a number of etiologies (see Table 20.1) [1, 2]. The degree and timing of the drop in platelets can be important clues for determining the etiology of thrombocytopenia. Heparin-induced thrombocytopenia (HIT) is an important consideration and is discussed in detail in Chap. 21. Other etiologies not specific to the perioperative setting should also always be considered including idiopathic thrombocytopenic purpura (ITP), sequestration, and malignancy-associated thrombocytopenia. Key data that should be gathered include:

M.B. Jackson et al. (eds.), *The Perioperative Medicine Consult Handbook*, DOI 10.1007/978-3-319-09366-6_20, © Springer International Publishing Switzerland 2015

TABLE 20.1 POTENTIAL ETIOLOGIES OF POSTOPERATIVE THROMBOCYTOPENIA

Etiology	Description
Consumption	Seen in larger blood loss surgeries Occurs immediately after surgery Returns toward normal within 2–3 days
Thrombocytopenia due to infection	Associated with both viral and bacterial infections Can be seen as part of disseminated intravascular coagulation (DIC) process Other mechanisms less well understood [1]
Pseudo-thrombocytopenia	Artifact due to EDTA in CBC tube. Clumping present on smear. Redraw platelet count in tube containing citrate instead of EDTA
Heparin-induced thrombocytopenia	Platelet count usually falls >50 % of baseline but nadirs >20,000/μL Can cause skin necrosis, DVT, pulmonary embolism, venous sinus thrombosis, and stroke (see Chap. 21)
Dilution of platelets after transfusion	Occurs soon after transfusion (may be soon after surgery if transfusions are given during case) Severity tends to be proportional to the volume of blood administered and usually seen in large volume resuscitations Clinical course usually benign Platelet count usually returns to normal within 3–5 days after blood transfusion [1]
Non-HIT drug-induced immune thrombocytopenia	Quinidine, digoxin, valproic acid, alpha-methyldopa, penicillin class drugs, thiazides, trimethoprim/sulfamethoxazole, cimetidine, famotidine Platelet count is often extremely low (can be less than 20,000) Can cause postoperative bleeding Platelet transfusions useful Steroids not shown to be useful [1]
Posttransfusion purpura	Acute thrombocytopenia caused by alloimmunization against transfused platelets occurs ~5–8 days after the transfusion Clinical presentation is similar in its severity to drug-induced immune thrombocytopenia with levels dropping below 20,000 and sudden onset of bleeding [1]

(continued)

Table 20.1 (CONTINUED)

Etiology	Description
Disseminated intravascular coagulation (DIC)	Can occur in the setting of severe infection as mentioned above
	Can also occur independent from infection after significant surgeries
	Often presents with an acute thrombocytopenia immediately after surgery
	Bleeding diathesis is more severe and more extensive than that which is expected from the degree of thrombocytopenia (because it is also associated with a coagulopathy) [1]
Thrombotic thrombocytopenic purpura (TTP)	Rare. Decreased platelets, increased LDH, normal PT/PTT [1]
	Classic pentad is fever, neurologic symptoms/altered mental status, renal failure, microangiopathic hemolytic anemia, and thrombocytopenia

- History: review medications (e.g., heparin), transfusion history, symptoms of infection, and symptoms/history of hematologic or liver disease
- Physical exam: assess for infection, splenomegaly, signs of liver disease, and evidence of thrombosis

Hematology consultation may be needed if no obvious etiology is found or if levels are low enough that platelet transfusion is considered. Consider the following studies in evaluation; however, send only those that are appropriate to the clinical situation (see Table 20.1):

- CBC with differential
- Reticulocyte count
- Haptoglobin, LDH, total and direct bilirubin
- PT/PTT/INR, fibrinogen, and peripheral smear
- Heparin-induced thrombocytopenia (HIT) panel

Monitoring/Prevention of Complications

- Intramuscular injections should be avoided in patients who are thrombocytopenic.
- Other drugs that interfere with platelet function (NSAIDs, aspirin, beta-lactam antibiotics) should generally be avoided depending on the indication.

- Platelet transfusions are usually indicated only for platelets <10,000 or <50,000 with active bleeding; this is important to discuss with the surgical team.

REFERENCES

1. George, J. Evaluation and management of thrombocytopenia by primary care physicians. In: UpToDate. Waltham, MA; Wolters Kluwer; 2012. http://www.uptodateonline.com. Last updated Nov 2013. Accessed Mar 2014.
2. Chang JC. Review: postoperative thrombocytopenia: with etiologic, diagnostic and therapeutic consideration. Am J Med Sci. 1996;311(2):96–105.

Chapter 21
Heparin-Induced Thrombocytopenia

Elizabeth Kaplan

BACKGROUND

Heparin-induced thrombocytopenia (HIT) is a recognized cause of perioperative complications, including skin necrosis, deep vein thrombosis (DVT), pulmonary embolism, venous sinus thrombosis, and stroke [1, 2]. HIT must be recognized in order to treat and prevent potentially catastrophic complications.

PERIOPERATIVE MANAGEMENT

WHEN TO SUSPECT HIT

HIT should be considered whenever a patient has unexplained thrombocytopenia. See Chap. 20 for discussion of a general approach to postoperative thrombocytopenia: platelet counts do not usually fall below 20,000 as a consequence of HIT, and other causes (drug-induced thrombocytopenia, disseminated intravascular coagulation, immune thrombocytopenic purpura, etc.) should be suspected if the platelet count is in this range [2]. Postoperative patients (particularly those with long spine or other major blood loss surgeries) often have depressed platelet counts for days postoperatively, but if the platelet count fails to rebound or falls 50 % or more from a baseline value, a diagnosis of HIT should be entertained [2]. Other red flags for HIT include [1, 2]:

- Thrombosis associated with thrombocytopenia
- Platelet count that has fallen 50 % or more from a baseline value (note that it may still be in the normal range)
- Necrotic skin lesions at heparin injection sites
- Prior exposure to heparin

M.B. Jackson et al. (eds.), *The Perioperative Medicine Consult Handbook*, DOI 10.1007/978-3-319-09366-6_21,
© Springer International Publishing Switzerland 2015

TABLE 21.1 TIMING OF PRESENTATIONS OF HIT

Early	Within the first 1–2 days of starting heparin	Seen in patients with prior exposure to heparin (usually in the preceding 3 months) and hence prior antibodies
Usual	Within 5–10 days of starting heparin therapy	Presumed to be due to the formation of new antibodies
Late	After discontinuation of heparin therapy. May be >2 weeks or more from last exposure to heparin	Can occur after the patient's discharge from the hospital. Suspect in a patient returning to the hospital with a new thrombotic complication, particularly after an orthopedic or other surgery where heparin prophylaxis was used

TYPICAL TIME COURSE OF THROMBOCYTOPENIA IN HIT

- Development of HIT varies depending on patients' prior exposure to heparin (and whether they already have antibodies) (see Table 21.1) [1, 2].
- A patient may present with HIT after stopping heparin.
- Nonimmune-mediated decrease in platelet count is seen in many patients within 2 days of starting heparin, but causes a lesser drop and will usually rebound despite continued heparin treatment [2].

EVALUATION

HIT is a clinical diagnosis, but certain lab tests are useful in supporting the diagnosis. HIT is caused by antibodies against the heparin/platelet factor 4 complex, and multiple tests are available to assess for the presence of these antibodies.

- The heparin antibody enzyme-linked immunosorbent assay (ELISA) is the most common test used; it is extremely sensitive but not specific.
- A negative ELISA can be useful in ruling out the diagnosis, but a positive test does not confirm it without further supporting features.
- We recommend first checking heparin antibody ELISA [3].
- If the ELISA is positive and there is a high clinical suspicion, then treat as HIT positive.
- If there is high clinical suspicion of false-positive, a serotonin release assay (SRA) can be checked [3].

TABLE 21.2 THE 4T'S PROBABILITY SCORE

Thrombocytopenia	Platelet count fall >50 % and nadir ≥20,000/µL	2 points
	Platelet count fall 30–50 % and nadir 10–19,000/µL	1 point
	Platelet count fall <30 % and nadir ≤10,000/µL	0 point
Timing of platelet fall	Clear onset between days 5 and 10 or platelet count fall at ≤1 day if with prior heparin exposure within the last 30 days	2 points
	Consistent with fall at 5–10 days but unclear onset after day 10, or fall ≤1 day with prior heparin exposure within 30–100 days	1 point
	Platelet count fall at <4 days without recent exposure	0 point
Thrombosis or other sequelae	Confirmed new thrombosis, skin necrosis, or acute systemic reaction after IV unfractionated heparin bolus	2 points
	Progressive or recurrent thrombosis, non-necrotizing skin lesions, or suspected thrombosis that has not been proven	1 point
	None	0 point
Other causes for thrombocytopenia present	None apparent	2 points
	Possible	1 point
	Definite	0 point

Test interpretation (total score from points above): 0–3, low probability; 4–5, intermediate probability; 6–8, high probability. Studies suggest using laboratory testing for HIT to patients with an intermediate or high 4T's pretest probability [3, 6]

There are multiple possible causes of postoperative thrombocytopenia. A pretest clinical score called "the 4T's" has been developed and prospectively validated to help determine who may benefit most from laboratory testing for HIT (see Table 21.2) [3–5]. This score may also be useful in interpreting tests based on pretest probability, especially if there is suspicion for a false-positive.

TREATMENT
- Stop all heparin products (including heparin flushes).
- Start a non-heparinoid anticoagulant (direct thrombin inhibitor bivalirudin or argatroban). Pharmacy protocols exist for this treatment and will vary from hospital to hospital.

- Start warfarin (only after non-heparinoid anticoagulant has been started) with a plan to anticoagulate for at least 6 weeks, but not until the patient's platelet count is greater than 100–150 K due to the risk of transient hypercoagulability.
- Therapy with warfarin should be overlapped for at least 5 days prior to discontinuation of the direct thrombin inhibitor.
- Hematology consultation may be very helpful when treating hospitalized patients with HIT.
- It is not recommended to re-challenge patients with heparin who have a history of HIT if other forms of anticoagulation are available. However, most patients with immune-mediated HIT lose their HIT antibodies within 3 months of ceasing therapy, and short-term heparin use (such as for cardiac bypass surgery) has been shown to be safe [7].
- Low-molecular-weight heparins (enoxaparin, dalteparin, etc.) and heparin analogues (fondaparinux) appear to have a lower risk of HIT and can be used when appropriate and after appropriate consideration of potential risks.

REFERENCES

1. Arepally G, Ortel T. Heparin-induced thrombocytopenia. N Engl J Med. 2006;355(8):809–17.
2. Coutre S. Heparin-induced thrombocytopenia. Topic update 12/17/12. In: Basow DS (ed) UpToDate. Waltham, MA; Wolters Kluwer; 2012. http://www.uptodateonline.com. Accessed Jan 2014.
3. University of Washington Medical Center Anticoagulation Services suggestions for clinical management of suspected heparin-induced thrombocytopenia (HIT). http://uwmcacc.org/pdf/VTE_HIT.pdf. Accessed 20 Dec 2013.
4. Lo GK, Juhl D, Warkentin TE, et al. Evaluation of pretest clinical score (4T's) for the diagnosis of heparin-induced thrombocytopenia in two clinical settings. J Thromb Haemost. 2006;4:759.
5. Cuker A, Gimotty PA, Crowther MA, Warkentin TE. Predictive value of the 4 Ts scoring system for heparin-induced thrombocytopenia: a systemic review and meta-analysis. Blood. 2012; 120:4160.
6. Bryant A, Low J, Austin S, Joseph JE. Timely diagnosis and management of heparin-induced thrombocytopenia in a frequent request, low incidence single centre using clinical 4T's score and particle gel immunoassay. Br J Haematol. 2008;143:721.
7. Follis F, Schmidt CA. Cardiopulmonary bypass in patients with heparin-induced thrombocytopenia and thrombosis. Ann Thorac Surg. 2000;70:2173–81.

Chapter 22
Anemia

Ronald Huang

BACKGROUND

Both preoperative and postoperative anemia are associated with increased morbidity and mortality after surgery [1–3]. The goals of managing anemia in the perioperative setting are identifying patients with anemia, optimizing hemoglobin and hematocrit, preventing unnecessary blood loss, and using red blood cell transfusions judiciously.

PREOPERATIVE EVALUATION

HISTORY AND PHYSICAL
- Ask about symptoms of anemia such as fatigue, exertional dyspnea, palpitations, lightheadedness, or angina.
- Gather a personal history of anemia, blood transfusions, bleeding (see Chap. 19), and chronic medical conditions that are known to result in anemia (e.g., chronic kidney disease, malignancy, rheumatoid arthritis).
- Physical exam may disclose signs of anemia (e.g., pallor, tachycardia) or may direct the examiner to suspect specific causes.

TESTING
- Hemoglobin and hematocrit, along with red blood cell indices, as part of a complete blood count (CBC), should be reviewed preoperatively when anemia is suspected based on the history and physical exam or when a significant amount of blood loss is expected with surgery.

M.B. Jackson et al. (eds.), *The Perioperative Medicine Consult Handbook*, DOI 10.1007/978-3-319-09366-6_22, © Springer International Publishing Switzerland 2015

- A routine CBC has also been recommended for patients older than 60 years old and patients with severe systemic disease (American Society of Anesthesiologists [ASA] class 3 or 4), although this recommendation is based on limited evidence [4].
- Hemoglobin and hematocrit are not indicated for young, healthy patients undergoing low-risk surgeries.
- If surgery is elective, unexplained anemia should be evaluated prior to surgery. The decision to delay surgery should take into account the urgency of the surgery, anticipated blood loss of the surgery, severity of the anemia, and suspected cause of anemia.
- Additional laboratory studies depend on the history and physical examination and CBC. These should include at least a repeat CBC, a reticulocyte count and peripheral blood smear along with either iron studies and ferritin for low mean corpuscular volume (MCV), creatinine for normal MCV, or vitamin B12 and folate for high MCV.

PERIOPERATIVE MANAGEMENT

TREATMENT OF PREOPERATIVE ANEMIA

- Treatment is directed toward causes of anemia that are easily reversible (e.g., iron, folate, or vitamin B12 deficiency) in a relatively short period of time (1–2 months) or that require attention prior to elective surgery (e.g., occult GI bleeding, malignancy).
- The treatment for iron deficiency anemia (low serum iron, high TIBC, low ferritin) is ferrous sulfate 325 mg BID to TID. Intravenous iron (ferric gluconate, iron sucrose) is available for patients who cannot tolerate or do not respond to oral preparations.
- The treatment for vitamin B12 deficiency is vitamin B12 1,000 mcg PO daily. Vitamin B12 is available in IM preparation for those who do not respond to oral supplementation.
- The treatment for folate deficiency is folate 1 mg PO daily.
- For each of the nutritional deficiencies, a reticulocyte count and CBC should be measured in 1 week to assess for response (reticulocytosis), then patients should have repeat CBC every month from their initial CBC until appropriate hemoglobin and hematocrit is achieved.

- A referral for endoscopy should be considered in patients with iron deficiency anemia, especially older patients.
- Pancytopenia or evidence of hemolysis (elevated reticulocyte count, abnormal peripheral smear, high LDH, low haptoglobin) should prompt a hematology consultation.
- Medications that may predispose the patient to bleeding should be discontinued or substituted.

TREATMENT OF INTRAOPERATIVE ANEMIA

- The intraoperative management of anemia is performed by anesthesia and surgical teams.
- The amount of blood loss can be estimated by direct visualization, using standard methods to quantify blood loss (e.g., suction devices), monitoring for physiologic changes of anemia, and laboratory studies. The amount of blood loss is often underestimated.
- Surgical technique and proper hemostasis are central to minimizing blood loss.
- Intraoperative anemia is primarily managed with allogenic red blood cell transfusion.
- Transfusion of autologous red blood cells collected preoperatively (preoperative autologous blood donation), immediately preoperatively (acute normovolemic hemodilution), or intraoperatively (red blood cell salvage) are less commonly employed options for patients who are unwilling to accept allogenic red blood cell transfusion. Preoperative autologous blood and red blood cell salvage (from surgical drains) are also used postoperatively.

INITIAL POSTOPERATIVE MANAGEMENT

- The postoperative evaluation of anemia begins with reviewing the operative report and anesthesia record for estimated blood loss and blood products administered during surgery. The medical consultant should assess the patient for ongoing blood loss, including surgical drains, and monitor for signs and symptoms of anemia.
- Not all patients require laboratory studies postoperatively. If there is significant intraoperative or ongoing postoperative blood loss or the patient is symptomatic or is at increased risk for bleeding, then a postoperative hemoglobin and hematocrit should be monitored.
- The postoperative management of anemia also involves preventing additional blood loss by taking careful consideration

TABLE 22.1 RECOMMENDATIONS FOR RED BLOOD CELL TRANSFUSION BASED ON HEMOGLOBIN [5–10]

Hgb < 7–8 g/dL—red blood cell transfusion is indicated
Hgb 8–10 g/dL—optimal transfusion threshold is unclear
Hgb > 10 g/dL—red blood cell transfusion is usually not necessary

Transfusion may be considered when the hemoglobin is between 8 and 10 g/dL, and there is ongoing or anticipated blood loss or there is clinical evidence of decreased tissue perfusion and oxygenation

prior to starting or resuming medications that predispose patients to bleeding, monitoring for and treating hemostatic abnormalities, treating underlying causes of anemia, and limiting the number and frequency of blood draws when appropriate (each vial is 2–10 mL).

■ Red blood cell transfusion is the treatment for severe postoperative anemia.

OPTIMAL TRANSFUSION THRESHOLD

■ Despite many studies to define the optimal threshold at which postoperative blood transfusion should be given, a definitive threshold has yet to be established [5–10].

■ The decision to transfuse depends mainly on a patient's hemoglobin or hematocrit, whether there are ongoing or anticipated blood losses, and how the patient is tolerating the degree of anemia. In the postoperative setting, studies in patients undergoing hip fracture repair and cardiac surgery support the use of a restrictive rather than a liberal transfusion strategy [7, 8]. Recommendations for red blood cell transfusion based on hemoglobin are listed in Table 22.1.

EFFECT OF RED BLOOD CELL TRANSFUSION

■ One unit of packed red blood cells (~300 mL) is expected to increase the hemoglobin by 1 g/dL or the hematocrit by ~3 % in an average 70 kg adult patient, if there is no active bleeding.

■ A posttransfusion hemoglobin or hematocrit can be sent as soon as 15 min following transfusion to assess for response.

RISKS OF TRANSFUSION

■ Red blood cell transfusions are associated with their own risks and costs [11–14]. The risks of transfusion include acute and delayed hemolytic reactions, febrile nonhemolytic reactions, allergic reactions, viral hepatitis and HIV, transfusion-related acute lung injury (TRALI), sepsis due to bacterial contamination, volume overload (or transfusion-associated circulatory overload [TACO]), and hyperkalemia.

- There remain concerns for other possible adverse effects, including potential exposure to emerging infectious agents, and immunomodulation from transfused blood that may predispose to bacterial infection [11, 12].

PATIENTS WHO DECLINE BLOOD TRANSFUSION

- Informed consent must be obtained prior to blood transfusion. Patients may decline transfusions for many reasons, most commonly for religious reasons (Jehovah's Witnesses).
- Typically, Jehovah's Witnesses do not accept whole blood or any of the "four major components" (i.e., red blood cells, platelets, plasma, and white blood cells). Many Jehovah's Witnesses also believe that blood should not be taken out of the body and stored for any length of time, and do not accept preoperative autologous blood donation.
- Patients who decline whole blood transfusion may or may not decide to accept certain medical therapy such as blood subfractions, recombinant coagulation factors, and autologous blood so long as it maintains a continuous circuit with their body.
- When caring for any patient who declines blood transfusion, it is important to respect the patient's decisions, establish a working relationship, maintain confidentiality, review the patient's understanding and personal position on medical therapy, and develop an appropriate blood management plan including a clear course of action if the worst-case scenario were to occur, and document carefully [15].
- Most of the strategies used for patients who decline blood transfusions are the same that are used for all patients to reduce the need for blood transfusion [16, 17]. Erythropoiesis-stimulating agents (see discussion below) and hemostatic agents (coagulation factors, antifibrinolytics, desmopressin, etc.) have more limited roles in the management of perioperative anemia.
- If there is a question whether care can be provided for such a patient, a referral should be considered. The Society for the Advancement of Blood Management, which is not affiliated with Jehovah's Witnesses, also maintains a list of hospitals in the United States with bloodless medicine and surgery programs (http://www.sabm.org).

ERYTHROPOIESIS-STIMULATING AGENTS

- Recombinant human erythropoietin (epoetin alfa) is FDA approved to reduce the need for blood transfusions in patient undergoing elective, noncardiac, nonvascular surgery.
- The benefit of epoetin alfa must be weighed against the potential risks of this therapy (death, myocardial infarction, stroke, deep vein thrombosis [DVT], and tumor progression).
- Depending on the timing of surgery, epoetin alfa may be given as 300 U/kg per day beginning 10 days before surgery, on the day of surgery, and for 4 days after surgery or it can be given as 600 U/kg once weekly 21, 14, and 7 days prior to surgery and on the day of surgery. Reticulocyte count will increase in the first few days. Hemoglobin increase varies but can be expected to rise by at least 1–2 g/L prior to surgery. Ferrous sulfate 325 mg PO daily should be given with epoetin alfa.
- Due to increased risk of DVT, DVT prophylaxis is recommended if epoetin alfa is given.

REFERENCES

1. Carson JL, Duff A, Poses RM, et al. Effect of anaemia and cardiovascular disease on surgical mortality and morbidity. Lancet. 1996;348(9034):1055–60.
2. Musallam KM, Tamim HM, Richards T, et al. Preoperative anaemia and postoperative outcomes in non-cardiac surgery: a retrospective cohort study. Lancet. 2011;378(9800): 1396–407.
3. Carson JL, Noveck H, Berlin JA, et al. Mortality and morbidity in patients with very low postoperative Hb levels who decline blood transfusion. Transfusion. 2002;42(7):812–8.
4. National Institute for Health and Care Excellence (NICE). Preoperative tests. The use of routine perioperative tests for elective surgery. Evidence, methods and guidance. Available at: http://www.nice.org.uk/nicemedia/live/10920/29094/29094.pdf
5. Hébert PC, Wells G, Blajchman MA, et al. A multicenter, randomized, controlled clinical trial of transfusion requirements in critical care. Transfusion Requirements in Critical Care Investigators, Canadian Critical Care Trials Group. N Engl J Med. 1999;340(6):409–17.
6. American Society of Anesthesiologists Task Force on Perioperative Blood Transfusion and Adjuvant Therapies. Practice guidelines for perioperative blood transfusion and adjuvant therapies: an updated report by the American Society of Anesthesiologists Task Force on Perioperative Blood Transfusion and Adjuvant Therapies. Anesthesiology. 2006;105(1): 198–208.
7. Hajjar LA, Vincent JL, Galas FR, et al. Transfusion requirements after cardiac surgery: the TRACS randomized controlled trial. JAMA. 2010;304(14):1559–67. doi:10.1001/jama.2010.1446.
8. Carson JL, Terrin ML, Noveck H, Sanders DW, Chaitman BR, Rhoads GG, FOCUS Investigators, et al. Liberal or restrictive transfusion in high-risk patients after hip surgery. N Engl J Med. 2011;365:2453–62.
9. Carson JL, Grossman BJ, Kleinman S, et al. Red blood cell transfusion: a clinical practice guideline from the AABB*. Ann Intern Med. 2012;157(1):49–58. doi:10.7326/0003-4819-157-1-201206190-00429.
10. Carson JL, Carless PA, Hebert PC. Transfusion thresholds and other strategies for guiding allogeneic red blood cell transfusion. Cochrane Database Syst Rev. 2012;4:CD002042. doi:10.1002/14651858.CD002042.pub3.
11. Goodnough LT, Brecher ME, Kanter MH, et al. Transfusion medicine. First of two parts—blood transfusion. N Engl J Med. 1999;340(6):438–47.

12. Klein HG, Spahn DR, Carson JL. Red blood cell transfusion in clinical practice. Lancet. 2007;370(9585):415–26.
13. Amin M, Fergusson D, Wilson K, et al. The societal unit cost of allogenic red blood cells and red blood cell transfusion in Canada. Transfusion. 2004;44(10):1479–86.
14. Varney SJ, Guest JF. The annual cost of blood transfusions in the UK. Transfus Med. 2003;13(4):205–18.
15. Rogers DM, Crookston KP. The approach to the patient who refuses blood transfusion. Transfusion. 2006;46(9):1471–7.
16. Goodnough LT, Shander A, Spence R. Bloodless medicine: clinical care without allogeneic blood transfusion. Transfusion. 2003;43(5):668–76.
17. Berend K, Levi M. Management of adult Jehovah's Witness patients with acute bleeding. Am J Med. 2009;122(12):1071–6. doi:10.1016/j.amjmed.2009.06.028.

Chapter 23
Sickle Cell Disease

Nason P. Hamlin

BACKGROUND

Patients with sickle cell disease (SCD) require special attention in the perioperative period. This is due, in part, to the physical properties of their abnormal hemoglobin(s) but also to comorbidities associated with SCD (e.g., anemia, functional asplenia, end-organ damage). The risk is higher for certain forms of SCD/thalassemia.

SCD patients also have special needs with regard to chronic pain control that can present additional challenges in the postoperative period.

Hospitals that regularly treat patient with sickle cell disease may have perioperative protocols to follow. For those without such protocols, what follows is an adaptation of a protocol used at the University of Washington/Seattle Cancer Care Alliance (SCCA). As such, it should be used as a basis for understanding some of the basic perioperative concerns for this special population rather than a mandated order set.

PREOPERATIVE EVALUATION

- Dental consult, if needed, for tooth removal and assessment of infection risk
- Nutrition consult, if needed, for nutrition lab screen, calorie needs evaluation, and supplements evaluation (see Chap. 41)
- End-organ screening for risk assessment and targeted management:
  - Transthoracic echocardiogram for TR jet velocity
  - PFT/6-min walk (see Chap. 27)
  - Urine protein and complete metabolic panel (CMP)

M.B. Jackson et al. (eds.), *The Perioperative Medicine Consult Handbook*, DOI 10.1007/978-3-319-09366-6_23, © Springer International Publishing Switzerland 2015

- Determine perioperative transfusion needs
- Check that the blood bank has RBC genotyping profile
- Confirm care plan with surgery, perioperative medicine consult, pain service, anesthesia, and hematology consult

PERIOPERATIVE MANAGEMENT

PREOPERATIVE MANAGEMENT

In many cases, the patient is admitted to the hematology service the day prior to surgery for preoperative optimization. Alternatively, the patient may be admitted to a surgical service with hematology or internal medicine consultation. Regardless, it is critical for several measures to be initiated preoperatively to both monitor the patient's hematologic status and decrease the chances of surgery precipitating a sickle cell vaso-occlusive crisis:

Two Days Prior to Surgery

- Check CBC/diff, reticulocyte count, quantitative hemoglobin S, type, and cross

One Day Prior to Surgery

- Check CBC/diff, CMP, magnesium, PT/PTT/INR/fibrinogen, and LDH
- Transfuse to hemoglobin 10 mg/dl using leukoreduced/antigen-matched blood products
- IV fluids: 1/2NS after transfusion at maintenance rate ($\approx$100 ml/h), add magnesium 8–16 m Eq/L if serum magnesium less than 2.2, and replete other electrolytes as needed
- Start incentive spirometry hourly while awake
- Confirm operative plan and suitability for postoperative transfer of the patient to the surgical service
- Confirm with blood bank that blood is available for surgery
- Confirm postoperative plan with pain service
- Consult hematology

INTRAOPERATIVE MANAGEMENT (THE PURVIEW OF THE ANESTHESIA TEAM)

- Confirm that preoperative antibiotics were given.
- Maintain oxygen $SaO_2 > 98$, $PaO_2 > 95$.
- Keep temperature >37: NO ICE (do not pack surgical site in ice). Use warmed IV fluids.

- Patients are very sensitive to volume overload and prone to pulmonary edema. Patients with high cardiac risk may benefit from intraoperative transesophageal echocardiography (TEE) monitoring.
- Use *hypotonic* IV fluids (e.g., 1/2NS, not NS or LR).

POSTOPERATIVE CARE

- Confirm that hematology consultant will see patient on POD 0
- Transfuse to keep Hgb 9–10/dl with leukoreduced/antigen-matched blood
- Avoid fluid overload
- Use *hypotonic* fluids (e.g., 1/2NS)
- Keep magnesium at the upper limits of normal (2.2–2.4)
- Avoid hypothermia—NO ICE
- Start incentive spirometry hourly while awake
- Avoid over sedation with narcotic analgesia (usually managed by the pain service)
- Early mobilization
- DVT prophylaxis with mechanical devices right away and anti-coagulant as soon as acceptable to the surgical team, preferably within 24 h (see Chap. 31)
- Continue outpatient medication, e.g., hydroxyurea and folate

Chapter 24
Cerebrovascular Disease

Anna L. Golob

BACKGROUND

Stroke is an uncommon but feared complication of surgery. The observed stroke rate is 0.3–3.5 % in general surgery patients, varying by age and other comorbidities [1]. Approximately one-third of postoperative strokes are embolic [2, 3]. A history of cerebrovascular disease is a risk factor for perioperative cerebrovascular and cardiovascular complications.

PREOPERATIVE EVALUATION

RISK STRATIFICATION: GENERAL CONSIDERATIONS

Prior stroke is a major risk factor: One retrospective surgical series of patients with a history of previous stroke found a 2.9 % incidence of postoperative stroke [4]. A case–control study found that history of previous stroke was the most significant risk factor for postoperative stroke [5]. Other possible risk factors include age (not independent, but as a marker of other cardiovascular disease), female gender, hypertension, diabetes, creatinine >2, smoking, chronic obstructive pulmonary disease, peripheral vascular disease, left ventricular ejection fraction <40 %, coronary artery disease, heart failure, and symptomatic carotid stenosis [2].

Medical consultants often evaluate patients who have had a recent cerebrovascular event being considered for surgery:

- Recommendations to delay elective surgery following a cerebrovascular accident (CVA) or transient ischemic attack (TIA) vary widely, from 2 weeks to 3 months [1].

M.B. Jackson et al. (eds.), *The Perioperative Medicine Consult Handbook*, DOI 10.1007/978-3-319-09366-6_24, © Springer International Publishing Switzerland 2015

- Each case should be individually evaluated with regard to the type and urgency of the surgery, the patient's comorbidities as a whole, and the extent to which the TIA/CVA symptoms are stable, have been fully evaluated, and intervened upon if appropriate (e.g., carotid endarterectomy [CEA] for recurrent TIA/CVA due to a carotid lesion).
- Patients whose stroke risk factors have been maximally treated without escalating symptoms are likely to be at lower risk.
- Discussion with the patient's neurologist regarding risk factor optimization is recommended.

PHYSICAL EXAMINATION

General cardiovascular examination and neurologic examination is indicated preoperatively for patients at risk for perioperative stroke [6]. If a carotid bruit is detected, the patient should be questioned for signs, symptoms, or history of TIA/CVA. Patients with truly asymptomatic, incidentally found carotid bruits do not require further workup prior to surgery:

- There is a poor correlation between asymptomatic bruits and significant carotid disease [7].
- Patients with known mild to moderate carotid stenosis have an overall low risk of perioperative stroke.
- A prospective study of 735 patients (excluding those with active symptoms) undergoing elective abdominal, cardiothoracic, breast, and extremity surgery failed to show a significant perioperative risk associated with asymptomatic carotid bruit on routine preoperative physical examination [8].

Indications for a carotid duplex in patients with a carotid bruit include:

- Symptomatic patients
- History of TIA/CVA
- Asymptomatic patients planned for coronary artery bypass grafting (CABG) given evidence for improved outcomes with combined CABG/CEA in patients found to have severe carotid stenosis [8]

PERIOPERATIVE MANAGEMENT

STROKE PREVENTION

There are no good data to support specific management strategies. We advise optimizing cardiovascular risk factors as possible, including blood pressure control, restarting medications such as aspirin and statins, and restarting anticoagulation when surgically acceptable with regard to bleeding risk. If the patient is anticoagulated due to high baseline stroke risk or prior CVA, consider bridging with unfractionated or low-molecular-weight heparin in the perioperative period (see Chaps. 9 and 18) [9]. Vigilance in detecting new-onset atrial fibrillation may reduce embolic disease.

POSTOPERATIVE STROKE

When a postoperative stroke does occur, it may be associated with mortality as high as 26 %, although estimates vary [3]. Management should proceed in the same way as a stroke not associated with a procedure. However, important considerations are the following [9]:

- Identify possible embolic sources.
- Work closely with the surgical team, should anticoagulation be indicated.
- Thrombolytics can be difficult to use because recent surgery is generally a contraindication; consider neurointerventional procedures in lieu of thrombolytics.
- "Permissive hypertension" may be difficult in certain vascular or plastic surgery procedures, and discussion with the surgery and neurology teams is essential. Hypotension should be avoided.
- Achieving normoglycemia and normal oxygenation and preventing fever remain important.
- Hyponatremia may be more difficult to avoid in the postoperative setting secondary to third spacing.

REFERENCES

1. Bell R, Merli G. Perioperative assessment and management of the surgical patient with neurologic problems. In: Merli G, Weitz H, editors. Medical management of the surgical patient. Philadelphia, PA: W. B. Saunders; 1998. p. 283.
2. Selim M. Perioperative stroke. N Engl J Med. 2007;356:706–13.
3. Parikh S, Cohen J. Perioperative stroke after general surgical procedures. N Y State J Med. 1993;93:162–5.
4. Landercasper J, Merz BJ, Cogbill TH, et al. Perioperative stroke risk in 173 consecutive patients with a past history of stroke. Arch Surg. 1990;125:986–9.
5. Limburg M, Wijdicks EF, Li H. Ischemic stroke after surgical procedures: clinical features, neuroimaging, and risk factors. Neurology. 1998;50:895–901.
6. Fleisher LA, Beckman JA, Brown KA, et al. ACC/AHA 2007 guidelines on perioperative cardiovascular evaluation and care for noncardiac surgery: a report of the American College of Cardiology/American Heart Association Task Force on Practice Guidelines. Circulation. 2007;116:e418–500.
7. Ropper AH, Wechsler LR, Wilson LS. Carotid bruit and the risk of stroke in elective surgery. N Engl J Med. 1982;307(22):1388–90.
8. Hines GL, Scott WC, Schubach SL, et al. Prophylactic carotid endarterectomy in patients with high-grade carotid stenosis undergoing coronary bypass: does it decrease the incidence of perioperative stroke? Ann Vasc Surg. 1998;12:23.
9. Szeder V, Torbey MT. Prevention and treatment of perioperative stroke. Neurologist. 2008;14(1):30–6.

Chapter 25
Epilepsy and Seizure Disorders

Tyler Lee

BACKGROUND

Patients with preexisting seizure disorder may have higher incidences of postoperative complications. Identification of these patients in the preoperative period is necessary to optimize perioperative management and minimize risk of seizure activity and associated complications [1].

PREOPERATIVE EVALUATION

Internal medicine consultants should consider the following when seeing patients with preexisting seizure disorders:

- Use of antiepileptic drugs (AEDs) and supplements, including dosages and adherence
- Presence of vagal nerve or other stimulators (discuss with neurology and anesthesia providers)
- Seizure type, frequency, and date of most recent seizure
- Perform a general neurologic examination to document any baseline abnormalities
- Most recent drug levels if indicated (usually not necessary to repeat levels if clinically stable or levels have been stable previously)
- Routine imaging or preoperative electroencephalography (EEG) usually not indicated

M.B. Jackson et al. (eds.), *The Perioperative Medicine Consult Handbook*, DOI 10.1007/978-3-319-09366-6_25,
© Springer International Publishing Switzerland 2015

PERIOPERATIVE MANAGEMENT

PATIENTS WITH PREEXISTING SEIZURE DISORDERS

Patients may be at increased risk for seizures in the perioperative period due to infection, electrolyte, and other metabolic disturbances. In a retrospective study, risk of seizures in the perioperative period was estimated between 1 and 5 % for patients with preexisting seizure disorders. Type of surgery or anesthesia was not associated with increased clinical seizure risk [2, 3]. Factors associated with increased risk of perioperative seizures include:

- More frequent preoperative seizures.
- Shorter time between the last seizure and surgery.
- Higher number of antiepileptic medications.
- When postoperative seizures do occur, they are typically the same phenotype as preoperative seizures [2].

Medication Management

Patients may be at increased perioperative risk of seizures because many AEDs can only be given PO (such as carbamazepine, gabapentin, lamotrigine, topiramate). Therefore, plan ahead if NPO status is anticipated postoperatively (Table 25.1). We recommend discussion with both pharmacy and neurology consultants if a patient's baseline medication needs to be switched to an alternative agent in IV form.

- In most cases, if the patient normally takes a morning dose of AED, that dose may be taken on the morning of surgery.
- If unable to take PO AEDs, use IV forms. Work with pharmacy and neurology consultants as needed. Transition to usual PO medications as soon as possible.
- Avoid hyponatremia. Monitor electrolytes if the surgical care is expected to produce alterations in electrolyte balance.
- Certain AEDs are associated with hyponatremia [4].

NEW-ONSET SEIZURES IN THE POSTOPERATIVE PERIOD

The exact incidence of postoperative seizures is unknown though cardiac and neurologic surgery is associated with higher risk. A broad differential diagnosis should be considered and the workup directed based on clinical suspicion. Neurology consultation may be warranted if etiology is unclear. Workup should include thorough history and physical, electrolytes, and evaluation for infection. Common etiologies include:

- Electrolyte abnormalities, especially sodium but also calcium and magnesium [5]

TABLE 25.1 COMMONLY USED ANTIEPILEPTIC MEDICATIONS AND ROUTES OF ADMINISTRATION

Medication	PO or IV	Notes
Phenytoin (Dilantin®)	PO, IV PO dose = IV dose	Commonly used antiepileptic medication for IV administration. Side effects include hypotension and arrhythmia when given IV (must be given slowly IV). Multiple drug interactions
Lamotrigine (Lamictal®)	PO	Few significant drug interactions. May lower oral contraceptive efficacy
Levetiracetam (Keppra®)	PO, IV	Few significant drug interactions
Valproic acid (Depakote®)	PO, IV	Recommend discussion with pharmacist or neurologist to convert from PO to IV. IV dosing uses valproate sodium. Drug interactions with azoles, warfarin
Phenobarbital	PO, IV	Recommend discussion with pharmacy to convert from PO to IV. Multiple drug interactions
Carbamazepine (Tegretol®)	PO	Multiple drug interactions
Zonisamide (Zonegran®)	PO	Few significant drug interactions
Topiramate (Topamax®)	PO	Some drug interactions at higher doses

- Medications (e.g., meperidine and carbapenem) may lower the seizure threshold
- Sepsis
- Withdrawal syndrome, such as from benzodiazepine or alcohol
- Central nervous system injury/intracranial surgery
- Stroke

REFERENCES

1. Chang CC, Hu CJ, Lam F, et al. Postoperative adverse outcomes in surgical patients with epilepsy: a population-based study. Epilepsia. 2012;53(6):987–94.
2. Niesen AD, Jacob AK, Aho LE, et al. Perioperative seizures in patients with a history of a seizure disorder. Anesth Analg. 2010;111(3):729–35.
3. Benish SM, Cascino GD, Warner ME, et al. Effect of general anesthesia in patients with epilepsy: a population-based study. Epilepsy Behav. 2010;17:87–9.
4. Grikiniené J, Volbekas V, Stakisaitis D. Gender difference of sodium metabolism and hyponatremia as an adverse drug effect. Medicina (Kaunas). 2004;40:935–42.
5. Castilla-Guerra L, et al. Electrolytes disturbances and seizures. Epilepsia. 2006;47(12):1990–8.

Chapter 26
Parkinson's Disease

Elizabeth Kaplan

BACKGROUND

Patients with Parkinson's disease are at increased risk for perioperative complications [1]. In a prospective study of perioperative complications, patients with Parkinson's disease were at significantly higher risk for all serious complications after correcting for other risk factors in a multivariate analysis (odds ratio 8.14, CI 1.76–37.67) [2]. Patients are generally thought to be at increased risk because of difficulty with mobility, swallowing, and decreased pulmonary reserve made worse if they miss medication doses in the perioperative period. These patients are also at increased risk for gastric dysmotility, orthostatic hypotension, delirium, and falls. There is no broad consensus statement or treatment guidelines for the perioperative approach to this disease [3]. However, many perioperative complications of Parkinson's disease can potentially be reduced by minimizing interruptions in Parkinson's disease medications [3].

PREOPERATIVE EVALUATION

Take a detailed history and perform an exam with particular focus on:

- Typical symptoms and signs related to the patient's Parkinson's disease
- Exact medication use including dosing and time of administration
- Typical reaction if the patient misses a dose [3]
- Whether the patient has a deep brain stimulator

Patients with Parkinson's tend to show a restrictive type picture on pulmonary function testing related to rigidity and bradykinesia of the respiratory muscles. In many patients this is improved by treatment

M.B. Jackson et al. (eds.), *The Perioperative Medicine Consult Handbook*, DOI 10.1007/978-3-319-09366-6_26, © Springer International Publishing Switzerland 2015

with levodopa [4]. It is important to be aware that patients may be at increased risk for perioperative pulmonary complications, but it is not necessary to routinely obtain pulmonary function tests (PFTs) before surgery. Alert the anesthesiologist if the patient has a deep brain stimulator as the anesthesiologist may need to plan for coordinating with the device's programmer to temporarily turn it off during surgery.

PERIOPERATIVE MANAGEMENT

MEDICATION MANAGEMENT

- Attempt to keep the timing of the patient's Parkinson's medication regimen the same as the outpatient regimen [3]. Patients may be very sensitive to the exact timing of their doses of some medications, including carbidopa/levodopa.
- Consult with the patient's outpatient neurologist about perioperative medication management.
- If the patient is expected to be NPO postoperatively, discuss with the patient's neurologist whether the patient should titrate medications down to the lowest possible dose prior to surgery [3].
- Carbidopa/levodopa and other medications can be given via nasogastric tube or percutaneous endoscopic gastrostomy (PEG) tube. Be aware that if the controlled release version of carbidopa/levodopa is crushed, it becomes 30 % more bioavailable and can cause an increased dose and toxicity.
- Be mindful of side effects and potential interactions of Parkinson's medications with typical perioperative medications (anesthetics, antiemetics, pain medications); these are summarized below for common Parkinson's medications [3].
- It is also good practice to consult with a pharmacist about potential drug interactions of new medications with patient's Parkinson's medications.

Carbidopa/Levodopa (Sinemet®)

- May precipitate confusion or hallucinations at higher doses and may increase the risk of urinary retention.
- Acute discontinuation of levodopa may rarely precipitate a neuroleptic malignant-like syndrome. It is best to taper the dose slowly.
- Some experts recommend reducing the dose of carbidopa/levodopa to the lowest possible preoperatively and then

resuming the drug postoperatively as soon as possible (to avoid the risks of abrupt discontinuation) [3].

MAO B Inhibitors: Selegiline (Eldepryl®), Rasagiline (Azilect®)

- Although designed to be a selective inhibitor of monoamine oxidase (MAO) type B, at higher doses (>10 mg) this drug does not act selectively.
- There are numerous drug interactions (at any dose), especially with meperidine and antidepressants (such as fluoxetine).
- At higher doses, interactions with sympathomimetic drugs and all narcotic analgesics are possible. Interactions can include serotonin syndrome.
- The traditional practice of discontinuing these medications 2 weeks prior to surgery may not be advisable in all patients with Parkinson's disease because of the risk of a flare of symptoms. Alternatively, it may not be possible to stop these drugs preoperatively in the case of urgent or emergent surgery. If it is not possible to stop these drugs before surgery, it is imperative to alert the anesthesiologist so that medications with higher risk (e.g., certain vasopressors) can be avoided [3].

Dopamine Agonists: Bromocriptine (Parlodel®), Pergolide (Permax®), Pramipexole (Mirapex®), Ropinirole (Requip®)

- These drugs can usually be given perioperatively, but use caution as they can cause postural hypotension and confusion.
- Occasionally held the evening before and the morning of surgery, and restarted postoperatively because of the risk of confusion, especially in the elderly patient.

COMT (Catechol-O-Methyltransferase Inhibitors): Entacapone (Comtan®) and Tolcapone (Tasmar®)

- These agents increase the plasma half-life of L-dopa and prolong the therapeutic effect of those medications.
- Typically can be continued perioperatively.
- May precipitate dyskinesias, hallucinations, confusion, and orthostatic hypotension [3].

MONITORING/PREVENTION OF COMPLICATIONS

- Patients who are unable to swallow their medications may be able to be managed with a feeding tube or a nasogastric (NG) tube, depending on the type of surgery they had and how long they are expected to not be able to take pills.

- If the patient is unable to take his or her usual medication by mouth for a prolonged period of time, consider neurology consultation to discuss conversion to intravenous alternatives.
- Avoid dopamine antagonists, including haloperidol, risperidone, metoclopramide, promethazine, and prochlorperazine, that are sometimes used in the postoperative period [1, 3]; these medications can worsen Parkinson's symptoms.
- Encourage general measures to improve pulmonary hygiene: incentive spirometry, elevating the head of the bed, and early mobilization. It is also important to institute measures designed to minimize the risk of delirium (see Chap. 46).
- Physical and occupational therapy may also prove beneficial perioperatively for transfers and routine activities of daily living (ADLs).
- Fall precautions.

REFERENCES

1. Brennan KA, Genever RW. Managing Parkinson's disease during surgery. BMJ. 2010;341: 990–3.
2. Reilly DF, McNeely MJ, Doerner D, et al. Self-reported exercise tolerance and the risk of serious perioperative complications. Arch Intern Med. 1999;159:2185–92.
3. Patel S, Stickrath C, Anderson M, Klepitaskaya O. How should Parkinson's disease be managed perioperatively? The Hospitalist, June 2010. http://www.the-hospitalist.org/details/article/704937/How_should_Parkinsons_disease_be_managed_perioperatively.html. Accessed 1 Dec 2011.
4. Sathyaprabha TN, Kapavarapu PK, Pall PK, et al. Pulmonary functions in Parkinson's disease. Indian J Chest Dis Allied Sci. 2005;47(4):251–7.

Chapter 27
Pulmonary Risk Assessment and Management

Sabeena Setia and John H. Choe

BACKGROUND

Postoperative pulmonary complications (PPCs) include atelectasis, bronchospasm, tracheobronchitis, pneumonia, pulmonary embolus, pneumonia, acute respiratory distress syndrome (ARDS), and respiratory failure. The reported incidence varies widely, with estimates ranging from 2 % up to 30 % of patients undergoing general anesthesia in different reports [1, 2]. Although greater attention is given to cardiovascular risk stratification, PPCs are likely more common and costly than cardiovascular complications and incur substantial morbidity and mortality [3]. Compared with cardiovascular risk stratification, fewer well-validated tools are available to predict PPCs. However, physicians need to be vigilant of the consequences and the prevention of postoperative pulmonary complications.

Asthma, chronic obstructive pulmonary disease (COPD), obstructive sleep apnea (OSA), and pulmonary hypertension are discussed separately (see Chaps. 28, 29, and 30).

PREOPERATIVE EVALUATION

Preoperative evaluation of all patients should include an assessment of risk factors for pulmonary complications; functional status is especially important to assess (see Table 27.1).

M.B. Jackson et al. (eds.), *The Perioperative Medicine Consult Handbook*, DOI 10.1007/978-3-319-09366-6_27,
© Springer International Publishing Switzerland 2015

TABLE 27.1 RISK FACTORS FOR PULMONARY COMPLICATIONS [1, 5]

COPD
Age > 60
ASA class II or higher
Functionally dependent
Congestive heart failure
Pulmonary hypertension
Delirium
Alcohol use
Obstructive sleep apnea
Albumin <3.6 g/dL
Surgery factors: prolonged surgery more than 3 h; site of surgery—abdominal, thoracic, neurosurgery, head and neck, and vascular surgery; emergent surgery; general anesthesia

ASA American Society of Anesthesiologists

- Although obesity alone is not associated with increased risk of PPCs, assessment of OSA risk and functional status are crucial in these patients [4].
- In patients with pulmonary hypertension, having New York Heart Association (NYHA) functional class >2, history of pulmonary embolism, or OSA increases the risk of PPCs [1].
- Echocardiography should be considered in patients with suspected heart failure as a cause of dyspnea.
- Albumin <3.6 g/dl predicts postoperative pulmonary complications. Surgeons are usually highly attentive to nutritional status for other reasons (overall morbidity, mortality, wound healing, etc.) and may delay surgery for those reasons. It is unclear if correction of hypoalbuminemia changes outcomes; generally, studies of perioperative nutritional supplementation (both enteral and parenteral) have been disappointing [5].
- Mild–moderate asthma has not been found to be a risk factor for postoperative pulmonary complications [1].
- Diagnostic tests such as a chest X-ray or pulmonary function tests, unless performed for new symptoms or an abnormal exam, often do not change perioperative management and should not be ordered unless there is a clinical indication (see Table 27.2).

TABLE 27.2 PREOPERATIVE PULMONARY DIAGNOSTIC TESTS

Chest X-ray	■ Routine pre-op chest X-rays are *not* indicated ■ No consensus—guidelines differ. ACP guidelines: "may be helpful" in patients >50 years of age who are undergoing upper abdominal, thoracic, or abdominal aortic aneurysm (AAA) surgery or in patients with cardiac or pulmonary disease [5]
Pulmonary function tests (PFTs)	■ Routine PFTs *not* indicated except for certain surgeries (e.g., thoracic surgery—usually defer this testing to the surgeon) ■ Known COPD: assess by symptoms and exam ■ Consider for patient with suspected but previously undiagnosed obstructive lung disease
Arterial blood gas (ABG)	■ Consider for patients with elevated serum HCO_3, O_2 dependence, moderate to severe COPD, or suspected obesity-hypoventilation syndrome

PERIOPERATIVE MANAGEMENT

PREOPERATIVE RECOMMENDATIONS

■ Advise smoking cessation. A meta-analysis concluded that the existing evidence does not support an increased risk of complications due to stopping smoking prior to surgery; the longer the period of smoking cessation, the greater the benefits [6].

■ The patient's home pulmonary medication regimen should be continued perioperatively, including both oral agents (e.g., montelukast) and inhaled agents (e.g., albuterol, ipratropium, and fluticasone).

■ Patients on long-term oral steroids may require supplemental stress dose steroids (see Chap. 14).

POSTOPERATIVE PULMONARY CARE

■ To prevent atelectasis, lung expansion maneuvers (e.g., incentive spirometry) are recommended by the American College of Physicians [5], but there is little convincing evidence of efficacy [7].

■ Nasogastric tubes to decrease aspiration risk should not be routinely used and are generally deferred to the surgical team [1, 5].

- Consider nocturnal oximetry in patients at high risk for hypoxemia (e.g., OSA, obesity-hypoventilation syndrome).
- Patients receiving mechanical ventilation should receive preventive measures against ventilator-associated pneumonia, which vary by protocol but typically include semi-upright bed positioning, daily sedation vacations, and a weaning plan.
- When asked to see a patient for hypoxemia, the medicine consultant should entertain a broad differential, including pulmonary edema, atelectasis, hypoventilation, pleural effusions, pneumonia, and pulmonary embolism.

REFERENCES

1. Bapoje SR, Whitaker JF, Schulz T, Chu ES, Albert RK. Preoperative evaluation of the patient with pulmonary disease. Chest. 2007;132:1637–45.
2. Rock P, Rich PB. Postoperative pulmonary complications. Curr Opin Anaesthesiol. 2003;16(2):123–31.
3. Shander A, et al. Clinical and economic burden of postoperative pulmonary complications: patient safety summit on definition, risk reducing interventions, and preventive strategies. Crit Care Med. 2011;39(9):2163–72.
4. Hong CM, Galvagno SM. Patients with chronic pulmonary disease. Med Clin North Am. 2013;97:1095–107.
5. Qaseem A, Snow V, Fitterman N, et al. Risk assessment for and strategies to reduce perioperative pulmonary complications for patients undergoing noncardiothoracic surgery: a guideline from the American College of Physicians. Ann Intern Med. 2006;144:575–80.
6. Mills E, Eyawo O, Lockhart I, et al. Smoking cessation reduces postoperative complications: a systematic review and meta-analysis. Am J Med. 2011;124:144–54.
7. Guimaraes MMF, El Dib RP, Smith AF, et al. Incentive spirometry for prevention of postoperative pulmonary complications in upper abdominal surgery. Cochrane Database Syst Rev. 2009;(3):CD006058 (updated 2011).

Chapter 28
Asthma and COPD

Sabeena Setia and John H. Choe

BACKGROUND

Patients with asthma and chronic obstructive pulmonary disease (COPD) have an increased risk of postoperative pulmonary complications including pneumonia, atelectasis, and respiratory failure [1]. However, mild to moderate asthma has not been shown to pose significant perioperative pulmonary risk [2]. For patients with known asthma or COPD, detailed examination and history are usually enough to assess severity; preoperative pulmonary function tests (PFTs) are useful only if obstructive lung disease is suspected but not previously documented.

PREOPERATIVE EVALUATION

- History and physical should focus on baseline exercise tolerance and any recent decline; triggers for asthma or COPD exacerbation; signs of active respiratory infection such as fever, purulent sputum, and worsening cough; and history of steroid use.
- PFTs with spirometry should be reserved for patients who are suspected of, but have not yet been diagnosed with, chronic obstructive pulmonary disease or asthma [2].
- Perform an electrocardiogram (ECG) in patients with severe COPD to assess for right heart strain.
- Consider an arterial blood gas (ABG) in patients suspected to have baseline CO_2 retention.
- Routine chest radiographs in patients with stable COPD or asthma are seldom helpful unless guided by symptoms or

M.B. Jackson et al. (eds.), *The Perioperative Medicine Consult Handbook*, DOI 10.1007/978-3-319-09366-6_28, © Springer International Publishing Switzerland 2015

physical examination findings suggestive of new or worsening disease [2]. However, bullous disease seen on a chest X-ray increases the risk of perioperative pneumothorax.

PERIOPERATIVE MANAGEMENT

PREOPERATIVE CONSIDERATIONS

- Delay purely elective surgery for patients with acute exacerbations of asthma or COPD.
- Recommend smoking cessation; start nicotine replacement therapy if indicated.
- Attention should be given to patients with steroid dependence, as they may need perioperative stress dose steroids (see Chap. 14).
- In general, the patient's home regimen should be continued perioperatively with the exception of theophylline. Although infrequently used, theophylline may complicate postoperative management due to its relatively narrow therapeutic window and potential for arrhythmias; recommend discussion with pulmonology [3, 4].
- All inhalers, including inhaled corticosteroids, should be used on the morning of surgery.

POSTOPERATIVE CONSIDERATIONS

- Consider scheduled nebulizers with albuterol and ipratropium in patients with COPD and prn treatment in patients with mild COPD who are not already on treatment.
- Although correct administration via metered dose inhaler can be equally effective, delivery via nebulizer or through the ventilator circuit may be necessary during the postoperative period.
- Postoperative use of epidural catheters for pain management may reduce the risk of pulmonary complications in patients with COPD [1, 5] and in general populations [6].
- Opiates should be minimized if possible due to risk of hypercarbia and hypoxia.
- Recommend aggressive pulmonary toilet and lung expansion maneuvers such as incentive spirometry (not specific to patients with obstructive lung disease; see Chap. 27). Lung expansion strategies can also include noninvasive positive-pressure ventilation for patients unable to participate in incentive spirometry.
- For patients that develop active exacerbations requiring corticosteroids, discuss with surgical team—steroids may impair wound healing. Assess for and treat hyperglycemia.

PERIOPERATIVE BETA-BLOCKERS IN ASTHMA/COPD PATIENTS

Systematic reviews have generally demonstrated that groups of patients with COPD or asthma who receive beta-blockers have no significant increase in symptoms or decrease in FEV1, even amongst patients with severe disease (FEV1 < 50 %) or positive bronchodilator response [7, 8]. For those rare individuals with history of previous adverse reactions to beta-blockers, the risk of COPD or asthma exacerbation must be weighed against the potential benefit of perioperative beta-blockade.

The above data pertain to all patients taking beta-blockers; there are insufficient data for beta-blockers strictly given for *perioperative* reasons, since most perioperative beta-blocker trials excluded patients with asthma. Note, however, that there are relatively few indications currently for initiation of perioperative beta-blockers (see Chap. 8).

REFERENCES

1. Smetana GW. Preoperative pulmonary evaluation. N Engl J Med. 1999;340:937–44.
2. Qaseem A, Snow V, Fitterman N, et al. Risk assessment for and strategies to reduce perioperative pulmonary complications for patients undergoing noncardiothoracic surgery: a guideline from the American College of Physicians. Ann Intern Med. 2006;144:575–80.
3. Qaseem A, Wilt TJ, Weinberger SE, American College of Physicians, American College of Chest Physicians, American Thoracic Society, European Respiratory Society, et al. Diagnosis and management of stable chronic obstructive pulmonary disease: a clinical practice guideline update from the American College of Physicians, American College of Chest Physicians, American Thoracic Society, and European Respiratory Society. Ann Intern Med. 2011;155: 179–91.
4. National Asthma Education and Prevention Program: Expert panel report III: Guidelines for the diagnosis and management of asthma. Bethesda, MD: National Heart, Lung, and Blood Institute; 2007 (NIH publication no. 08-4051). www.nhlbi.nih.gov/guidelines/asthma/asthgdln.htm. Accessed Jan 2012.
5. van Lier F, van der Geest PJ, Hoeks SE, van Gestel YR, Hol JW, Sin DD, Stolker RJ, Poldermans D. Epidural analgesia is associated with improved health outcomes of surgical patients with chronic obstructive pulmonary disease. Anesthesiology. 2011;115(2):315–21.
6. Pöpping DM, Elia N, Marret E, Remy C, Tramèr MR. Protective effects of epidural analgesia on pulmonary complications after abdominal and thoracic surgery a meta-analysis. Arch Surg. 2008;143(10):990–9.
7. Salpeter SR, Ormiston TM, Salpeter EE. Cardioselective beta-blockers for chronic obstructive pulmonary disease. Cochrane Database Syst Rev. 2005;(4) Art. No.: CD003566. doi:10.1002/14651858.CD003566.pub2 (updated August 2010).
8. Salpeter SR, Ormiston TM, Salpeter EE, Wood-Baker R. Cardioselective beta-blockers for reversible airway disease. Cochrane Database Syst Rev. 2002; (4). Art. No.: CD002992. doi: 10.1002/14651858.CD002992 (updated June 2011).

Chapter 29
Obstructive Sleep Apnea and Obesity Hypoventilation Syndrome

Molly Blackley Jackson and Karen A. McDonough

BACKGROUND

Sleep-disordered breathing affects approximately 20 % of adults and is even more common among patients preparing for surgery [1]. Seven percent of adults have moderate or severe obstructive sleep apnea (OSA). A small subset of these patients suffer from obesity hypoventilation syndrome (OHS), defined as awake hypoventilation in the setting of obesity and sleep-disordered breathing [2]. The prevalence of OHS is 0.15–0.3 % in adults, but up to 8 % in patients preparing for bariatric surgery [3–5].

OSA is a major risk factor for intra- and postoperative complications, including hypoxemia, hypercarbia, unplanned reintubation, pneumonia, all-cause respiratory failure, cardiac complications (arrhythmia, myocardial injury), ICU transfer, and longer length of stay [6–8]. Patients with OHS are more likely to have pulmonary hypertension (PAH) than those with simple OSA and are at even higher risk for complications, including increased risk for heart failure and angina, need for invasive mechanical ventilation, and need for long-term care at discharge [3, 9]. Perioperative sleep deprivation and use of sedative/analgesic medications likely contribute to these risks.

In patients with OSA, a few small studies have shown that compliance with continuous positive airway pressure (CPAP) preoperatively and immediately postoperatively is associated with fewer postoperative complications [10, 11].

M.B. Jackson et al. (eds.), *The Perioperative Medicine Consult Handbook*, DOI 10.1007/978-3-319-09366-6_29, © Springer International Publishing Switzerland 2015

PREOPERATIVE EVALUATION

Along with focused preoperative history/physical examination, screen all preoperative patients with an OSA screening tool, such as STOP-BANG (see Table 29.1) [12].

- Consider OSA in patients with STOP-BANG score of ≥3.
- Consider OHS in patients with STOP-BANG score of ≥3 and a serum bicarbonate ≥28 and/or room air hypoxia (SpO$_2$ < 90 %).
- In patients with suspected OSA or OHS with elevated serum bicarbonate, consider preoperative arterial blood gas (ABG) to clarify baseline degree of hypercarbia.
- If you suspect OSA in a patient undergoing major elective surgery, refer for overnight polysomnogram (PSG).

The American College of Chest Physicians recommends against routine evaluation for pulmonary hypertension in patients with OSA [13]. However, consider a transthoracic echocardiogram (TTE) in the following cases:

- Suspicion of heart failure by history or exam (rales, S3, elevated jugular venous pressure)
- Suspicion of PAH by history, exam (loud P2, RV heave), or ECG (right axis deviation, right bundle branch block) (see Chap. 30)
- Patient with (or at risk for) OHS, who will undergo major surgery
- Patient with newly diagnosed severe OSA, who will undergo high-risk surgery and/or is likely to receive high doses of postoperative opioids

TABLE 29.1 STOP-BANG SCREENING TOOL [12]

S = Snoring. Do you snore loudly (louder than talking or loud enough to be heard through closed doors)?

T = Tired. Do you often feel tired, fatigued, or sleepy during daytime?

O = Observed (apnea). Has anyone observed you stop breathing during your sleep?

P = Pressure. Do you have (or are you being treated for) high blood pressure?

B = BMI > 35 kg/m^2

A = Age > 50 years old

N = Neck circumference > 40 cm

G = Male gender

High risk of OSA: ≥3 yes
Low risk of OSA: <3 yes

PERIOPERATIVE MANAGEMENT

PREOPERATIVE MANAGEMENT

- Ascertain and document CPAP or bilevel positive airway pressure (BPAP) settings, type of mask, amount of bleed-in oxygen (if any), and actual patient compliance.
- If patients have an ill-fitting mask, refer back to sleep clinic for mask refitting.
- Remind patients to bring their mask and machine to the hospital.
- Recommend good compliance with CPAP/BPAP preoperatively.
- Alert anesthesia and operative team to OSA or OHS diagnosis; these teams may consider regional anesthesia or peripheral nerve block to minimize sedation.

POSTOPERATIVE MANAGEMENT

- After major surgery, consider ICU care, depending on extent of surgery, severity of OSA/OHS, and compliance with CPAP/BPAP.
- Keep head of bed elevated ($\geq 30°$), or use lateral (side-lying) position [1].
- Extubate to CPAP or BPAP at home settings, and continue with naps and overnight sleep.
- Minimize the use of sedatives and opiate analgesics (considering scheduled acetaminophen or NSAIDS to augment pain control in appropriate candidates).
- Consider hypercarbia (and ABG) in patients with unexpected postoperative sedation or confusion.
- Close respiratory monitoring with continuous oximetry, especially in patients on sedating medications.
- If cannot tolerate CPAP/BPAP (or cannot use due to surgical site), initiate supplemental O2 (exercise caution in patients with concomitant COPD).
- For patients with OSA undergoing ambulatory or same-day surgery, American Society of Anesthesiologists guidelines recommend observing for an additional 3 h before discharge home, and if any episode of airway obstruction or apnea, monitoring should continue for additional 7 h [13, 14].

REFERENCES

1. Adesanya AO, Lee W, Greilich NB, Joshi GP. Perioperative management of obstructive sleep apnea. Chest. 2010;138(6):1489–98.
2. Olson A, Zwillich C. The obesity hypoventilation syndrome. Am J Med. 2005;118:948–56.

3. Nowbar S, Burkart KM, Gonzales R, et al. Obesity-associated hypoventilation in hospitalized patients: prevalence, effects, and outcome. Am J Med. 2004;116:1–7.
4. Chau E, Lam D, Wong J, et al. Obesity hypoventilation syndrome: a review of epidemiology, pathophysiology, and perioperative considerations. Anesthesiology. 2012;117:188–205.
5. Frey WC, Pilcher J. Obstructive sleep-related breathing disorders in patients evaluated for bariatric surgery. Obes Surg. 2003;13:676–83.
6. Kaw R, Pasupuleti V, Walker E, Ramaswamy A, Foldvary-Schafer N. Postoperative complications in patients with obstructive sleep apnea. Chest. 2012;141:436–41.
7. Memtsoudis S, Liu SS, Ma Y, et al. Perioperative pulmonary outcomes in patients with sleep apnea after noncardiac surgery. Anesth Analg. 2011;112:113–21.
8. Chung SA, Yuan H, Chung F. A systematic review of obstructive sleep apnea and its implications for anesthesiologists. Anesth Analg. 2008;107:1543–63.
9. Berg G, Delaive K, Manfreda J, Walld R, Kryger MH. The use of health-care resources in obesity-hypoventilation syndrome. Chest. 2001;120:377–83.
10. Gupta RM, Parvizi J, Hanssen AD, Gay PC. Postoperative complications in patients with obstructive sleep apnea syndrome undergoing hip or knee replacement: a case-control study. Mayo Clin Proc. 2001;769:897–905.
11. Rennotte MT, Baele P, Aubert G, Rodenstein DO. Nasal continuous positive airway pressure in the perioperative management of patients with obstructive sleep apnea submitted to surgery. Chest. 1995;1072:367–74.
12. Chung F, Yegneswaran B, Liao P, et al. STOP questionnaire: a tool to screen patients for obstructive sleep apnea. Anesthesiology. 2008;108(5):812–21.
13. Atwood Jr CW, McCrory D, Garcia JG, Abman SH, Ahearn GS, American College of Chest Physicians. Pulmonary artery hypertension and sleep-disordered breathing: ACCP evidence based clinical practice guidelines. Chest. 2004;126:72S–7.
14. Gross JB, et al. Practice guidelines for the perioperative management of patients with obstructive sleep apnea: an updated report by the American Society of Anesthesiologists Task Force on Perioperative Management of Patients with Obstructive Sleep Apnea. Anesthesiology. 2014;120(2):268–86.

Chapter 30
Pulmonary Hypertension

Brian S. Porter

BACKGROUND

Pulmonary hypertension (PH) confers increased risk of perioperative morbidity and mortality for patients undergoing noncardiac surgery [1–6]. Surgery in patients with PH can result in hypoxia, hypercapnia, and volume shifts exacerbating the underlying pulmonary hypertension, leading to acute right ventricular failure. Pathophysiologic effects may quickly spiral out of control as pulmonary pressures rise, causing worsening cardiac output, systemic hypotension, cardiac ischemia, and ultimately death.

Management of patients with pulmonary hypertension undergoing cardiac surgery is a complex subject outside the scope of this chapter. Consultation with a cardiac anesthesiologist is recommended in such cases.

PREOPERATIVE EVALUATION

Prospective identification of patients at high risk of poor surgical outcomes is difficult due to a paucity of published data. For the same reason, quantitative risk stratification is impossible. Additionally, recent expert consensus statements do not provide recommendations for the perioperative management of such patients [7, 8]. Given these challenges, the medical consultant can play a valuable role by providing preoperative risk estimates based on sound clinical judgment and by providing thoughtful management expertise postoperatively.

M.B. Jackson et al. (eds.), *The Perioperative Medicine Consult Handbook*, DOI 10.1007/978-3-319-09366-6_30, © Springer International Publishing Switzerland 2015

PATIENTS WITHOUT KNOWN PULMONARY HYPERTENSION

A careful history, physical examination, and review of the medical record should be performed. Abnormal findings associated with occult pulmonary hypertension include:

- Symptoms: exercise intolerance, dyspnea
- Comorbid disease states: chronic obstructive pulmonary disease (COPD), obesity, obstructive sleep apnea, left heart disease, connective tissue disease, chronic thromboembolic disease
- Signs: unexplained hypoxia, elevated neck veins, pedal edema, tricuspid regurgitation murmur, loud P2
- ECG: right axis deviation or right bundle branch block [9]
- CXR: wide pulmonary arteries, cardiomegaly
- PFTs: decreased diffusing capacity of lung for carbon monoxide (DLCO)

If there is clinical suspicion for pulmonary hypertension, echocardiography can provide an estimate of pulmonary artery (PA) pressure and is the preferred initial test [10]. Pulmonary artery catheterization can measure the hemodynamic variables required for a formal diagnosis (mean resting PA pressure ≥ 25 mmHg), but is invasive, expensive, and typically reserved for patients with known PH.

PATIENTS WITH KNOWN PULMONARY HYPERTENSION

There are different etiologies of pulmonary hypertension [10, 11], and chronic therapy varies with the underlying cause. However, with respect to surgical risk, it is unknown whether etiology is an important factor [5]. Given this uncertainty, it is reasonable to use the same risk stratification algorithm on all patients with PH, regardless of underlying cause.

The primary goal of the preoperative consultation for patients with known PH is to determine disease severity. Mild pulmonary hypertension confers limited additional surgical risk, but severe disease appears to markedly increase the perioperative risk of death or major adverse outcome, including stroke, myocardial infarction, heart failure, or arrhythmia [1, 3, 12, 13].

Determination of Disease Severity

The consultant should estimate functional capacity as measured by the World Health Organization (WHO) class (modified New York Heart Association functional class) [14]:

- Class I: no physical limitations
- Class II: mild limitation
- Class III: major limitations
- Class IV: completely unable to perform physical activities without symptoms and may be dyspneic at rest

Additional useful tests include:

- Echocardiogram within prior 12 months, with assessment of right ventricular function and estimation of mean or systolic PA pressure
- 6-minute walk distance (optional) [15]
- PA catheterization (optional, but encouraged in high-risk situations)

The history should be correlated with test results to estimate the current severity of the patient's disease. Although echocardiogram reports often include an estimate of disease severity based on the measured PA pressure, there are no strict definitions of mild, moderate, or severe disease states. Good clinical judgment is necessary. Generally, patients without symptoms and with only slightly abnormal normal test results have mild disease. Patients with slight functional impairment and somewhat abnormal test results have moderate disease. Patients with symptoms at rest and grossly abnormal test results have severe disease.

Several conditions may independently increase a patient's surgical risk in the setting of pulmonary hypertension and should be recognized if present:

- Decompensated cirrhosis [12, 16]
- Pregnancy coexisting with right ventricular dysfunction [17]
- History of pulmonary embolism [1]
- Planned thoracic surgery or orthopedic surgery [1]
- Emergency surgery [4, 13]

Ultimately, the disease severity, awareness of the patient's comorbid conditions, and knowledge of the planned procedure can be correlated to produce a qualitative overall estimate of the patient's surgical risk as shown in Table 30.1.

PERIOPERATIVE MANAGEMENT

SURGICAL PLANNING AND INTRAOPERATIVE CONSIDERATIONS

Detailed intraoperative planning is best left to the anesthesiologist and surgeon working in conjunction with the patient's pulmonary hypertension specialist. However, the following strategies may reduce surgical risk:

- Avoid emergency surgery if possible [3, 13].
- Use open rather than laparoscopic surgery, which may prolong anesthesia time and cause hypercarbia [3].
- Regional anesthesia may be safer than general anesthesia [6, 13].
- Split longer complex cases into shorter, lower-risk procedures [3, 13].

TABLE 30.1 RISK STRATIFICATION AND SUGGESTED PERIOPERATIVE MANAGEMENT STRATEGIES FOR PATIENTS WITH PULMONARY HYPERTENSION

Severity of pulmonary hypertension	Comorbid features associated with increased risk[a]	Estimated surgical risk	Suggested management strategy
Severe disease ■ WHO class III/IV ■ mPAP >55 ■ PASP >60 ■ 6-minute walk: <150 m	One or more	High	*Elective surgery:* avoid surgery if possible *Emergency surgery:* obtain cardiac anesthesiology and PH specialist consultation. Consider palliative care or another nonsurgical option. Proceed to surgery with caution if other alternatives are not possible
Moderate disease ■ WHO class II ■ mPAP 41–55 ■ PASP 45–59 ■ 6-minute walk: 150–400 m	One or more	Medium	*Elective surgery:* if patient's pulmonary hypertension has not been optimized through medical management or other means, or if etiology is unclear, then defer surgery. However, if etiology is known, the disease is stable, and no further improvement in severity is expected to occur, then proceed to surgery cautiously. *Emergency surgery:* proceed with surgery cautiously. Consider cardiac anesthesiologist consultation
Mild disease ■ WHO class I ■ mPAP 26–40 ■ PASP <45 ■ 6-minute walk: >400 m	None	Low	*Elective surgery:* proceed with surgery cautiously *Emergency surgery:* not applicable (patients undergoing emergency surgery should be considered to be at medium or high risk in most cases)

[a]Decompensated cirrhosis, pregnancy with RV failure, history of PE, thoracic surgery, orthopedic surgery, emergency surgery

MEDICATION MANAGEMENT

If a patient is being treated with prostacyclins or vasodilators, dosing of these agents should be left to the discretion of the treating anesthesiologist and the patient's pulmonologist or cardiologist. In many cases the patient's baseline therapy is continued and vasodilators are used in addition as needed.

Patients who are receiving treatment to control the underlying cause of the pulmonary hypertension should continue this treatment through the perioperative period in most cases (e.g., bronchodilators for COPD).

Some patients with pulmonary hypertension are treated with chronic anticoagulation. Unless the patient is receiving therapy for a separate indication, such patients probably do not require perioperative bridging with heparin. Postoperatively, patients should receive standard venous thromboembolic (VTE) prophylaxis until bleeding risk is acceptable, at which point anticoagulation may be resumed.

MONITORING AND PREVENTING POSTOPERATIVE COMPLICATIONS

Patients with severe pulmonary hypertension and those requiring intraoperative vasopressors should receive initial postoperative care in an ICU setting [1]. Attention to the following principles may reduce postoperative risk:

Optimize Volume Status

- Volume status should be meticulously monitored and optimized as necessary [1, 18].
- Patients coming from the operating room may have received significant volumes of intravenous fluid, putting them at risk for acute right heart failure; aggressive diuresis may be required in such cases.

Minimize Hypoxia

- Even low-risk patients may have occult nocturnal hypoxia [19], which could be particularly dangerous in the perioperative setting. Adequate oxygenation should be diligently maintained throughout the entire postoperative period.
- Consider the use of a continuous pulse oximeter during the first 48 h postoperatively when patients are likely to require sedatives or narcotics and the risk of morbidity is particularly high.

Optimize Analgesia

- Maintaining excellent analgesia postoperatively can help avoid dangerous increases in pulmonary pressure [6].
- However, respiratory depression can also exacerbate pulmonary hypertension, so narcotics must be used judiciously.
- Local anesthetics, NSAIDs, and nonpharmacologic analgesia strategies may be preferred.

REFERENCES

1. Ramakrishna G, Sprung J, Ravi BS, et al. Impact of pulmonary hypertension on the outcomes of noncardiac surgery: predictors of perioperative morbidity and mortality. J Am Coll Cardiol. 2005;45(10):1691–9.
2. Kaw R, Sharma P, Minai OA. What risks does a history of pulmonary hypertension present for patients undergoing noncardiac surgery? Cleve Clin J Med. 2007;74 Suppl 1:S20–1.
3. Lai HC, Lai HC, Wang KY, et al. Severe pulmonary hypertension complicates postoperative outcome of non-cardiac surgery. Br J Anaesth. 2007;99(2):184–90.
4. Memtsoudis SG, Ma T, Chiu YL, et al. Perioperative mortality in patients with pulmonary hypertension undergoing major joint replacement. Anesth Analg. 2010;111(5):1110–6.
5. Kaw R, Pasupuleti V, Deshpande A, et al. Pulmonary hypertension: an important predictor of outcomes in patients undergoing non-cardiac surgery. Respir Med. 2011;105(4):619–24.
6. Minai OA, Yared J, Kaw R, et al. Perioperative risk and management in patients with pulmonary hypertension. Chest. 2013;144(1):329–40.
7. Fleisher LA, Beckman JA, Brown KA, et al. ACC/AHA 2007 guidelines on perioperative cardiovascular evaluation and care for noncardiac surgery: a report of the American College of Cardiology/American Heart Association Task Force on Practice Guidelines. Circulation. 2007;116:e418–500.
8. McLaughlin VV, Archer SL, Badesch DB, et al. ACCF/AHA 2009 expert consensus document on pulmonary hypertension. J Am Coll Cardiol. 2009;53:1573–619.
9. Poirier P, Alpert MA, Fleisher LA, et al. Cardiovascular evaluation and management of severely obese patients undergoing surgery: a science advisory from the American Heart Association. Circulation. 2009;120:86–95.
10. McLaughlin VV, McGoon MD. Pulmonary arterial hypertension. Circulation. 2006;114(13):1417–31.
11. Simonneau G, Galiè N, Rubin L, et al. Clinical classification of pulmonary hypertension. J Am Coll Cardiol. 2004;43:5–12.
12. Krowka MJ, Plevak DJ, Findlay JY, et al. Pulmonary hemodynamics and perioperative cardiopulmonary-related mortality in patients with portopulmonary hypertension undergoing liver transplantation. Liver Transpl. 2000;6(4):443–50.
13. Price LC, Montani D, Jaïs X, et al. Noncardiothoracic nonobstetric surgery in mild-to-moderate pulmonary hypertension. Eur Respir J. 2010;35(6):1294–302.
14. Humbert M, Sitbon OS, Simmoneau G. Treatment of pulmonary arterial hypertension. N Engl J Med. 2004;351:1425–36.
15. ATS Committee on Proficiency Standards for Clinical Pulmonary Function Laboratories. ATS statement: guidelines for the six-minute walk test. Am J Respir Crit Care Med. 2002;166(1):111–7.
16. Collisson EA, Nourmand H, Fraiman MH, et al. Retrospective analysis of the results of liver transplantation for adults with severe hepatopulmonary syndrome. Liver Transpl. 2002;8(10):925–31.
17. Jones AM, Howitt G. Eisenmenger syndrome in pregnancy. Br Med J. 1965;1(5451):1627–31.
18. Rodriguez R, Pearl RG. Pulmonary hypertension and major surgery. Anesth Analg. 1998;87(4):812–5.
19. Minai O, Budev MM. Treating pulmonary arterial hypertension: cautious hope in a deadly disease. Cleve Clin J Med. 2007;74(11):789–806.

Chapter 31
Venous Thromboembolic Disease

Elizabeth Kaplan

BACKGROUND

Venous thromboembolism (VTE) is a known possible complication of surgical procedures. In early studies, the incidence of fatal pulmonary embolism, in the absence of prophylaxis, was estimated to be 0.1–0.8 % in patients undergoing elective general surgery, 2–3 % in patients having elective total hip replacement, and 4–7 % of patients undergoing surgery for a fractured hip [1, 2]. The risk for VTE in surgical patients is determined by the combination of patient-related predisposing factors (discussed below) and the specific type of surgery (time length of immobilization, degree of invasiveness, time of postoperative hospitalization) [2]. Evidence-based guidelines have been published for VTE prevention as well as for management of patients currently receiving anticoagulation for prior deep vein thrombosis (DVT) or pulmonary embolism (PE) in the perioperative period [1, 3–5]. The risk of new or recurrent VTE versus the risk of perioperative bleeding while on anticoagulation should be discussed with the surgeon so that a multidisciplinary decision can be made about perioperative anticoagulation management.

PREOPERATIVE EVALUATION

PATIENTS WITHOUT KNOWN VTE
- Factors which increase risk for perioperative VTE: malignancy, hereditary thrombophilias, pregnancy, prolonged immobility, and certain surgical procedures, including abdominal, gynecologic, orthopedic spine, and lower extremity surgery.

M.B. Jackson et al. (eds.), *The Perioperative Medicine Consult Handbook*, DOI 10.1007/978-3-319-09366-6_31,
© Springer International Publishing Switzerland 2015

- Medication management to reduce risk of perioperative VTE: hormone replacement therapy or oral contraceptives (with careful discussion of other contraceptive options) should be stopped if possible (see Chap. 4).
- Imaging: there are no data to support screening imaging studies prior to surgery in asymptomatic patients.

PATIENTS RECEIVING ANTICOAGULATION FOR PRIOR VTE

Recommendations differ regarding the perioperative management of patients who are receiving anticoagulation for a prior VTE. However, the perioperative consultant should consider the following:

- In general, the closer in proximity to the venous thromboembolic event, the higher the risk of a recurrent event in the perioperative period.
- Purely elective procedures should be avoided within the first month following a VTE and should be discouraged within the first 3 months.
- If it is determined that surgery should proceed while patient is still receiving treatment for VTE with warfarin, bridging therapy should be considered to minimize the time of therapy required during the perioperative period.

All decisions about anticoagulation management must be individualized for a patient's particular risk of both VTE and surgical bleeding (Table 31.1) [1, 6–9]. There are various bridging protocols in use; if it is determined bridging therapy is indicated (see Chap. 18 for examples of bridging protocols). There is practice variation regarding the use of IV heparin or therapeutic-dose low-molecular-weight heparin (LMWH) for bridging off and back on to warfarin. IV heparin has the advantage of reversibility and remains a useful postoperative option. Its disadvantage, especially preoperatively, is that it requires administration in the hospital. Note that LMWH should be avoided in patients with a CrCl <30. Work with the patient's pharmacist or use IV heparin if bridging therapy is indicated in patients with markedly reduced renal function. After surgery, anticoagulation may be restarted when surgical bleeding risk is acceptable, usually at least 48–72 h post-op. A 24-h interval may be acceptable for low-bleeding-risk surgery per American College of Chest Physicians (ACCP) guidelines, but should be discussed with the surgical team.

Use of Rivaroxaban

- Rivaroxaban has recently been approved for treatment of acute thromboembolism (DVT or PE). Perioperative management of this agent should be discussed with a pharmacist.

TABLE 31.1 MANAGEMENT OF PATIENTS WITH PRIOR VTE IN THE PERIOPERATIVE PERIOD [3–6]

Time of VTE prior to surgery	Risk of recurrent VTE after stopping anticoagulation	Management	
		Pre-op	Post-op
Within 1 month	Approaches 50 % if stopped prior to 1 month	Avoid surgery if possible Bridge from warfarin with IV heparin or LMWH Consider IVC filter	Bridge with IV heparin or LMWH
1–3 months prior	Risk decreases sharply after 1 month At 1 month ≈ 8 % At 3 months ≈ 4 %	Delay surgery if possible Consider bridge therapy from warfarin with IV heparin or LMWH	Bridge with IV heparin or LMWH
>3 months prior	3 months of anticoagulation is a reasonable amount of time prior to surgery	No bridging unless severe hypercoagulable state is present Most patients will have completed VTE therapy after 3 months—if they are still receiving anticoagulation, there is usually an additional risk factor or indication	Prophylaxis-dose LDUH or LMWH until on therapeutic anticoagulation Consider bridging with IV heparin or therapeutic-dose LMWH if severe hypercoagulable state

Notes: If a patient is hospitalized and not receiving bridge therapy, then prophylaxis-dose LDUH or LMWH should be given

Patients with a creatinine clearance <30 ml/min should not receive LMWH for bridge therapy but instead should receive IV unfractionated heparin. Management of patients being treated for acute VTE with an agent other than warfarin or heparin should be discussed with pharmacy

LDUH low-dose unfractionated heparin, *LMWH* low-molecular-weight heparin

- Rivaroxaban dosing in general should be reduced in patients with impaired renal function (based on creatinine clearance) and not used in patients with creatinine clearance <30 mg/dl [8].
- The medication should be held at least 24–48 h prior to surgery depending on the risk of bleeding in the procedure, the patient's age, and their renal function [6, 8].

Consideration of Inferior Vena Cava Filters

The function of an inferior vena cava (IVC) filter is to provide a mechanical interruption in the vena cava to prevent major pulmonary embolism. Anticoagulation is still indicated once surgical bleeding risk is low enough. Data on the use and efficacy of filters are scant. Possible indications for IVC filters are the following:

- Acute proximal DVT with an absolute contraindication to therapeutic anticoagulation due to bleeding [3]
- Acute VTE within 2 weeks of surgery and high risk of bleeding while on IV heparin [2, 10]
- Large PE and poor baseline cardiopulmonary reserve such that another embolic event would be poorly tolerated (even if able to be anticoagulated) [11]

Potentially retrievable IVC filters may be considered when the contraindication to anticoagulation is likely to be temporary (e.g., <2 weeks). Ability to remove a filter decreases with time—retrieval should generally occur by 3 months [12, 13]. A time course for possible retrieval should always be discussed with the proceduralist.

PERIOPERATIVE MANAGEMENT

The main concerns for perioperative management are prevention of VTE in all patients, resumption of anticoagulation in those patients who are chronically receiving it, and diagnosis and treatment of new postoperative VTE.

VTE PROPHYLAXIS FOR ALL PATIENTS

VTE prophylaxis recommendations are shown in Table 31.2. The suggested types of prophylaxis for each type of surgery are based on the 2012 ACCP guidelines [4, 5], which do not make specific dose recommendations for all methods of pharmacologic prophylaxis. Specific dosing recommendations (e.g., for LMWH) are further derived from the University of Washington Department of Pharmacy Anticoagulation Services website [8]. Be aware that decisions regarding

TABLE 31.2 RECOMMENDED VTE PROPHYLAXIS [5, 12, 13]

Type of surgery	First line	Second line	Notes
Orthopedic surgery			
Hip replacement (THA), knee replacement (TKA), hip fracture surgery (HFS)	LMWH (enoxaparin 30 mg SC q 12 h or dalteparin 5,000 U SC once daily) Start ≥ 12 h pre-op, and give the first post-op dose after ≥12 h post surgery Treatment duration: minimum 10–14 days	LDUH, fondaparinux, warfarin, aspirin, IPC Treatment duration: minimum 10–14 days	Treated duration recommended to extend for up to 35 days ACCP guidelines "suggest" LMWH in preference to the other options. With the exception of fondaparinux, the second-line options listed may not be as effective Use of aspirin alone remains controversial Consider IPC in addition to pharmacologic while hospitalized If increased bleeding risk: IPC or no prophylaxis Newer anticoagulants (THA, TKA only): see text
Knee arthroscopy	No prophylaxis		
General surgery, abdomen/pelvis surgery			
Very low risk <0.5 % (e.g., ambulatory same-day surgery)	Early ambulation		
Low risk ~1.5 % (e.g., certain laparoscopic procedures, more minor abdominal, gynecologic, urologic procedures)	IPC		

(continued)

TABLE 31.2 (CONTINUED)

Type of surgery	First line	Second line	Notes
Moderate risk ~3 % (e.g., major abdominal, nonmalignant gynecologic, thoracic, cardiac surgery)	LMWH, LDUH	IPC	Use IPC if high risk for major bleeding or if consequences of bleeding would be particularly severe
High risk ~6 % (e.g., abdominal/gynecologic malignancy surgery, bariatric (see below for bariatric specifics))	LMWH, LDUH +/−ES/IPC Extend duration if abd/pelvic cancer surgery	IPC	Use IPC if high risk for major bleeding or if consequences of bleeding would be particularly severe. If bleeding risk diminishes, add back pharmacologic prophylaxis If cannot use LMWH or LDUH, and not at high risk of bleeding, can use low-dose aspirin (160 mg), fondaparinux, or IPC
Bariatric	LMWH high-dose prophylaxis (e.g., enoxaparin 40 mg SC q 12 h for BMI >40) +/−IPC	LDUH +/−IPC	Consult with clinical pharmacist for weight-based dosing. Consider higher doses of LDUH if this option is chosen
Cardiac surgery	IPC		If prolonged hospital course due to non-hemorrhagic complications, add LDUH or LMWH

(continued)

TABLE 31.2 (CONTINUED)

Type of surgery	First line	Second line	Notes
Thoracic surgery	Moderate risk of VTE: LDUH, LMWH can add ES/IPC if high risk of VTE	Moderate risk of VTE: IPC	If high risk of bleeding, use IPC
Craniotomy	IPC		If high risk of VTE, add pharmacologic prophylaxis once bleeding risk is acceptable
Spinal surgery	IPC	LMWH, LDUH	If high risk for VTE, add pharmacologic prophylaxis once bleeding risk is acceptable
Major trauma	LDUH, LMWH, or IPC		IVC filter not recommended

LDUH = low-dose unfractionated heparin, dosing usually 5,000 U SC Q8H or Q12H

LMWH = low-molecular-weight heparin, suggested dosing listed in the above table

IPC = intermittent pneumatic compression, Warfarin is dose adjusted to an INR 2–3

LMWH = low-molecular-weight heparin, e.g., enoxaparin 40 mg SC once daily unless otherwise noted, dalteparin 5,000 U SC once daily

LDUH = low-dose unfractionated heparin, typically 5,000 U Q8H or Q12H

IPC = intermittent pneumatic compression

ES = elastic stockings, recommended 18–23 mmHg at the ankle [13]

timing and method of prophylaxis are usually at the discretion of the surgeon with consideration to the risk of surgical bleeding. For further dose-related questions, one should discuss with a clinical pharmacist. In general, the current guidelines favor individualized assessment taking into account both patient risks and surgical risks of VTE [5].

Considerations

- *Aspirin*: The American Academy of Orthopedic Surgeons guidelines allow for the use of aspirin 325 mg BID as prophylaxis [14]. The ACCP guidelines now accept this as an option for orthopedic surgery, although there is still controversy regarding its use [4, 15].
- For orthopedic surgery, the fondaparinux, rivaroxaban, and warfarin options may have increased bleeding risk compared to the other methods [4].
- *Neuraxial anesthesia*: The use of neuraxial anesthesia may complicate the use of LMWH and warfarin [8]. Generally use low-dose unfractionated heparin (LDUH) instead.
- *Body weight*: Dose adjustment of LMWH is often needed in the very obese (e.g., the bariatric surgery patient) and those with very low body weight.
- *Chronic kidney disease:* For VTE prophylaxis, dalteparin does not typically need dose adjustment. However, other LMWH such as enoxaparin may need dose adjustment or additional monitoring with factor Xa levels.
- *Vascular surgery*: Unless other risk factors are present, no pharmacologic prophylaxis is recommended. Most patients receive either heparin or antiplatelet agents.
- *Burns*: If there are additional risk factors (advanced age, morbid obesity, extensive or lower extremity burns, lower extremity trauma, femoral venous catheter, prolonged immobility), then use LMWH or LDUH when surgically acceptable.

Role of Newer Oral Anticoagulants

- Fondaparinux, a factor Xa inhibitor, has been approved in the USA for VTE prophylaxis in patients undergoing hip fracture surgery, hip replacement surgery, knee replacement surgery, or abdominal surgery [4, 5, 16].
- Dabigatran, a direct IIa (thrombin) inhibitor, has been approved in the USA for stroke prevention in atrial fibrillation. It has also been studied for VTE prophylaxis in patients undergoing hip and knee arthroplasty and for treatment of acute VTE, demonstrating efficacy comparable to enoxaparin and warfarin, respectively; however, it has not been yet approved, as of this writing, in the USA for these indications.
- Rivaroxaban, a direct Xa inhibitor, has been approved in the USA for VTE prophylaxis in those undergoing knee or hip arthroplasty.

- Both dabigatran and rivaroxaban are renally metabolized and may need dose reduction in those with at least moderate renal impairment.
- Apixaban, another direct Xa inhibitor, has been approved in Europe for VTE prophylaxis following knee and hip arthroplasty but is still undergoing further study in the USA as of this writing [17].
- According to the ACCP guidelines, newer anticoagulants may be considered for patients who decline injections. However, the long-term safety is unknown, and only rivaroxaban currently has FDA approval for VTE prophylaxis.

PATIENTS WITH PRIOR VTE REQUIRING ANTICOAGULATION

- Resume anticoagulation as described in Table 31.1, with close consultation with the patient's surgeon with regard to timing and bleeding risk.
- Until therapeutic-dose anticoagulation has been resumed postoperatively, prophylactic-dose pharmacologic VTE prophylaxis should be considered if the bleeding risk is acceptable.
- The timing of warfarin re-initiation depends on the assessment of bleeding risk. ACCP guidelines recommend resuming warfarin approximately 12–24 h after surgery if there is adequate hemostasis [6].

ACUTE POSTOPERATIVE VTE

Despite best efforts, postoperative VTE still occurs. Patients may present with acute hypoxia, dyspnea, tachycardia, and limb edema. Keep in mind that patients in the postoperative state may have other explanations for symptoms of VTE, so clinical suspicion remains vital so that VTE is not missed. Screening in asymptomatic patients is not recommended. Diagnostic testing for suspected postoperative VTE is shown in Table 31.3.

Immediate Management

- Immediate management consists of stabilization of the patient. Severity of the VTE and risk of bleeding must be assessed. Treat with therapeutic-dose anticoagulation as soon as possible. It is critical to discuss bleeding risk with surgery team. If anticoagulation is not an option due to bleeding risk, then an IVC filter may be considered (see above discussion on filters). See Table 31.4 for potential options.
- Thrombolytics are indicated for massive PE (SBP < 90) [18]. Contraindications include intracranial neoplasm, history of

TABLE 31.3 DIAGNOSTIC TESTING FOR SUSPECTED POSTOPERATIVE VTE

Test	Notes
Chest CT, PE protocol	Requires 18 gauge antecubital IV, Power PICC™, or PowerPort™ to deliver an adequately timed contrast bolus for the study to be properly interpreted Uses IV contrast—caution in patients with kidney disease
V/Q scan	Consider if contraindication to CT May be difficult to interpret in patients with underlying lung disease
Lower extremity duplex	Use if suspected DVT or if suspected PE and unable to perform chest CT or V/Q scan A single negative lower extremity duplex does not rule out PE
D-dimer	Not used—generally not useful in post-op patients, who may have elevated values due to other reasons and in whom low values would not preclude further evaluation for VTE

TABLE 31.4 STRATEGIES FOR MANAGEMENT OF POSTOPERATIVE VTE

Bleeding risk	Management of DVT/PE
Anticoagulation unacceptable	IVC filter until able to anticoagulate Consider potentially retrievable IVC filter Give prophylactic-dose unfractionated heparin or LMWH if possible
Anticoagulation acceptable, but high risk	IV heparin. Consider using "no-bolus" protocol
Anticoagulation acceptable, low risk	IV heparin or LMWH (therapeutic dose), then begin warfarin

intracranial hemorrhage/hemorrhagic stroke, and internal bleeding within 6 months. Due to bleeding risk, this option must always be discussed with the surgeon.

■ Catheter embolectomy is an option in centers with appropriate expertise for patients with massive PE [7, 18].
■ For upper extremity and catheter-associated DVT, current recommendations favor treating with LMWH, IV heparin, or fondaparinux [19]. In the postoperative setting, choice of anticoagulant must consider bleeding risk and reversibility.

Choice of Anticoagulation Agent

- IV heparin and LMWH have been found to be equal in efficacy for treatment of acute VTE. A systematic review found that LMWH had a significant reduction in thrombotic complications, hemorrhage, and mortality compared to unfractionated heparin in patients with DVT [20]. However, IV heparin may be advantageous postoperatively because of its short half-life and is reversible.
- Rivaroxaban has recently been approved for treatment of VTE, but caution should be used in patients with renal dysfunction; it should be avoided in patients with creatinine clearance <30 mg/dl.
- Fondaparinux has also been approved for the initial treatment of acute VTE as a bridge to warfarin [16].

SUBACUTE AND LONG-TERM MANAGEMENT

- For acute VTE, administer IV heparin/LMWH for at least 5 days total and until the INR is ≥2.0 for at least 24–48 h (i.e., usually need to give additional heparin after the first INR is in target range).
- If using dalteparin as an LMWH agent, dosing is typically 200 U/kg SC daily. Discuss with a clinical pharmacist for dose adjustments that may need to be made for CrCl < 30, weight >98 kg, and pregnancy. Enoxaparin dosing is typically 1 mg/kg SC BID and similar dose adjustments may be necessary, particularly for CrCl < 30.
- Consider LWMH alone if VTE is in association with malignancy [21]. However, cost is a concern.
- Duration of therapy for VTE is often 3 months if there was a reversible, transient risk factor (e.g., recent surgery, immobilization) [19].
- Duration of therapy is at least 3 months for unprovoked VTE. After 3 months, risk–benefit of further anticoagulation should be assessed. For a proximal DVT with low bleeding risk and close monitoring while on anticoagulation, long-term therapy is recommended. For a second unprovoked VTE, long-term therapy is also recommended [6, 19].
- Use compression stockings for DVT to reduce the risk of post-thrombotic syndrome.

REFERENCES

1. Geerts WH, Pineo GF, Heit JA, Bergqvist D, Lassen MR, Colwell CW, Ray JG. Prevention of venous thromboembolism: the seventh ACCP conference on antithrombotic and thrombolytic therapy. Chest. 2004;126(3 Suppl):338S.
2. Pai M, et al. Prevention of venous thromboembolic disease in surgical patients. UptoDate. Article revision date 3/2014. Accessed Mar 2014.
3. Kearon C, Kahn SR, Agnelli G, et al. Antithrombotic therapy for venous thromboembolic disease. Chest. 2008;133:454–545.
4. Falck-Ytter Y, Francis CW, Johanson NA, Curley C, Dahl OE, Schulman S, et al. Prevention of VTE in orthopedic surgery patients. Antithrombotic therapy and prevention of thrombosis, 9th ed: American College of Chest Physicians Evidence-Based Clinical Practice Guidelines. Chest. 2012;141(2 Suppl):e278S–325.
5. Gould MK, Garcia DA, Wren SM, Karanicolas PJ, Arcelus JI, Heit JA, et al. Prevention of VTE in nonorthopedic surgical patients: antithrombotic therapy and prevention of thrombosis, 9th ed: American College of Chest Physicians Evidence-Based Clinical Practice Guidelines. Chest. 2012;141:e227S–77.
6. Lip G. Management of anticoagulation before and after elective surgery. UptoDate. Article revision date 10/2013. Accessed Jan 2014.
7. Kearon C, Hirsh J. Management of anticoagulation before and after elective surgery. N Engl J Med. 1997;336:1506–11.
8. University of Washington Department of Pharmacy Anticoagulation Services. www.uwm-cacc.org. Last update Nov 2013. Accessed Jan 2014.
9. Douketis JD, Spyropoulos AC, Spencer FA, Mayr M, Jaffer AK, Eckman MH, et al. Perioperative management of antithrombotic therapy. Chest. 2012;141 (2 Suppl):e326S–50.
10. Geerts WH, et al. http://www.tigc.org/clinical-guides/Inferior-Vena-Cava-Filters.aspx. Accessed May 2011, Jan 2014.
11. Fedullo P, et al. Placement of inferior vena cava filters and their complications. UptoDate. Article revision date Oct 2013. Accessed Jan 2014.
12. Imberti D, Biachi M, Farina A, et al. Clinical experience with retrievable vena cava filters: results of a prospective observational multicenter study. J Thromb Haemost. 2005;3:1370–5.
13. Mismetti P, Rivron-Guillot K, Quenet S, et al. A prospective long-term study of 220 patients with a retrievable vena cava filter for secondary prevention of venous thromboembolism. Chest. 2007;131:223–9.
14. American Academy of Orthopaedic Surgeons—Medical Specialty Society. 2007 May. American Academy of Orthopaedic Surgeons clinical guideline on prevention of symptomatic pulmonary embolism in patients undergoing total hip or knee arthroplasty. http://www.ngc.gov/content.aspx?id = 10850. Accessed Dec 2011.
15. Stewart D, Freshour J. Aspirin for the prophylaxis of venous thromboembolic events in orthopedic surgery patients: a comparison of the AAOS and ACCP guidelines with review of the evidence. Ann Pharmacother. 2013;47(1):63–74.
16. US Food and Drug administration Drug Database. FDA/Center for Drug Evaluation and Research. Office of Communications, Division of Online Communications. http://www.accessdata.fda.gov/scripts/cder/drugsatfda/index.cfm?fuseaction=Search.Search_Drug_Name. Update frequency: Daily. Accessed Jan 2014.
17. Galanis T, Thomson L, Palladino M, et al. New oral anticoagulants. J Thromb Thrombolysis. 2011;31(3):310–20.
18. Jaff MR, McMurtry S, Archer SL, et al. Management of massive and submassive pulmonary embolism, iliofemoral deep vein thrombosis, and chronic thromboembolic pulmonary hypertension: a scientific statement from the American Heart Association. Circulation. 2011;123:1788–830.
19. Kearon C, Aki EA, Comerota AJ, Prandoni P, Bounameaux H, Goldhaber SZ, et al. Antithrombotic therapy for VTE disease. Antithrombotic therapy and prevention of thrombosis, 9th ed: American College of Chest Physicians Evidence-Based Clinical Practice Guidelines. Chest. 2012;141:e419S–94.

20. Erkens PM, Prins MH. Fixed dose subcutaneous low molecular weight heparins versus adjusted dose unfractionated heparin for venous thromboembolism. Cochrane Database Syst Rev. 2010 Sep 8;(9):CD001100.
21. Lee AY, Levine MN, Baker RI, et al. Low-molecular-weight heparin versus a coumarin for the prevention of recurrent venous thromboembolism in patients with cancer. N Engl J Med. 2003;349:146–5.

Chapter 32
Restrictive Lung Disease

Nina Saxena

BACKGROUND

Restrictive lung disease (RLD) is highly prevalent, frequently disabling, and is caused by a myriad of both pulmonary and extrapulmonary conditions (see Table 32.1) [1]. It is defined as a reduction of total lung capacity (TLC) below the 5th percentile of the predicted value, with a preserved one second forced expiratory volume to forced vital capacity ratio (FEV1/FVC) [1, 2, 3, 4]. The diffusion capacity of carbon monoxide (DLCO) can help distinguish between RLD due to intrinsic lung disease, in which DLCO is frequently reduced, and extrapulmonary restriction, in which DLCO is preserved [2, 5]. Because of the difficulty in diagnosis and variety of etiologies, the clinical impact of RLD is not well understood [1, 6]. Patients with RLD are thought to be at risk for exaggerated postoperative pulmonary complications, although the degree of risk has not been well studied [7, 8]. Underlying restrictive deficits may be worsened by perioperative atelectasis, loss of inspiratory muscle tone during anesthesia, pulmonary edema, or postoperative pneumonia [7].

PREOPERATIVE EVALUATION

EVALUATION OF PATIENTS WITH KNOWN RLD

- There are no evidence-based recommendations for the preoperative evaluation of patients with RLD.
- The management of patients with RLD depends upon the underlying etiology. For example, obesity may also be associated with sleep-disordered breathing and should be evaluated as such (Chap. 29). Other diseases, such as sarcoidosis and

M.B. Jackson et al. (eds.), *The Perioperative Medicine Consult Handbook*, DOI 10.1007/978-3-319-09366-6_32, © Springer International Publishing Switzerland 2015

TABLE 32.1 CAUSES OF RESTRICTIVE LUNG DISEASE [1, 7]

Pulmonary causes
  Atelectasis
  Pulmonary edema
  Acute respiratory distress syndrome
  Interstitial lung diseases
  Connective tissue diseases
  Vasculitis, granulomatous diseases, hypersensitivity pneumonias
  Drug-related pulmonary fibrosis
  Radiation therapy
  Lung resection
Extrapulmonary causes
  Obesity
  Skeletal/costovertebral deformities (e.g., scoliosis)
  Neuromuscular disorders (e.g., amyotrophic lateral sclerosis)
  Sternal deformities (e.g., pectus excavatum)
  Phrenic nerve injuries
  Pneumothorax

hypersensitivity pneumonitis, can have concomitant airway hyperreactivity and should be treated similarly to chronic obstructive pulmonary disease (Chap. 28) [7].

- As with all patients with pulmonary disease, evaluation should include a detailed history of functional status and other risk factors for postoperative pulmonary complications (Chap. 27) [9].
- Consider an arterial blood gas, as this may be useful in estimating perioperative oxygenation and ventilation needs [7, 10].
- A chest X-ray is only useful in patients with acute dyspnea or if comparison studies are available to monitor for progression of disease [7, 10].
- Spirometry is not useful unless concomitant undiagnosed obstruction is suspected [8].

EVALUATION OF PATIENTS SUSPECTED OF HAVING RLD

- The symptoms of RLD are nonspecific and patients generally present with dyspnea and cough [1]. A careful history should assess for mobility, dyspnea on exertion, and other markers of fitness [9].
- Chest radiographs are generally only useful for evaluating acute dyspnea. CT scans are only indicated if tracheal compression or other pathologic conditions are suspected [7, 10].

- Spirometry is useful as an initial assessment of lung function, but more detailed PFTs, including lung volumes and DLCO, are necessary to diagnose restriction and can give further insight as to the underlying cause [2, 3, 5].
- Consider an arterial blood gas in patients with O2 dependence or severe dyspnea as this may help predict perioperative oxygenation and ventilation [7, 10].

POSTOPERATIVE MANAGEMENT

- There are no evidence-based guidelines for the postoperative management of RLD.
- Recommendations are based on the underlying etiology of disease and a pulmonary consult is warranted in patients with severe respiratory compromise.
- Management should focus on preventing atelectasis, pulmonary edema, postoperative pneumonia, and muscle weakness as these can worsen underlying restrictive deficits [7].
- Lung expansion techniques may prevent atelectasis and are recommended by the ACP. Data suggest they are superior to no prophylaxis in preventing postoperative pulmonary complications in all patients undergoing abdominal surgery, although no modality of expansion showed clear superiority (Chap. 27) [8].
- As with all pulmonary diseases, maintenance of adequate nutrition and selective use of nasogastric decompression after abdominal surgery are important in preventing complications [8, 10].

REFERENCES

1. Scarlata S, Costanzo L, Giua R, Pedone C, Incalzi RA. Diagnosis and prognostic value of restrictive ventilatory disorders in the elderly: a systematic review of the literature. Exp Gerontol. 2012;47(4):281–9. doi:10.1016/j.exger.2012.02.001.
2. Pellegrino R, Viegi G, Brusasco V, et al. Interpretative strategies for lung function tests. Eur Respir J. 2005;26(5):948–68. doi:10.1183/09031936.05.00035205.
3. Glady CA, Aaron SD, Lunau M, Clinch J, Dales RE. A spirometry-based algorithm to direct lung function testing in the pulmonary function laboratory. Chest. 2003;123(6):1939–46.
4. Barreiro TJ, Perillo I. An approach to interpreting spirometry. Am Fam Physician. 2004;69(5):1107–14.
5. Bernstein W. Pulmonary function testing. [Miscellaneous Article]. Curr Opin Anaesthesiol. 2012;25(1):11–6. doi:10.1097/ACO.0b013e32834e7ad2.
6. Brown KK, Schwarz MI. Classifying interstitial lung disease: Remembrance of things past. Chest J. 2006;130(5):1289–91. doi:10.1378/chest.130.5.1289.
7. Hong CM, Galvagno Jr SM. Patients with chronic pulmonary disease. Med Clin North Am. 2013;97(6):1095–107. doi:10.1016/j.mcna.2013.06.001.

8. Qaseem A, Snow V, Fitterman N, et al. Risk Assessment for and Strategies To Reduce Perioperative Pulmonary Complications for Patients Undergoing Noncardiothoracic Surgery: A Guideline from the American College of Physicians. Ann Intern Med. 2006;144(8):575–80. doi:10.7326/0003-4819-144-8-200604180-00008.
9. Dronkers JJ, Chorus AMJ, van Meeteren NLU, Hopman-Rock M. The association of pre-operative physical fitness and physical activity with outcome after scheduled major abdominal surgery. Anaesthesia. 2013;68(1):67–73. doi:10.1111/anae.12066.
10. Simić D, Ladjević N, Milenović M, Bogićević A, Strajina V, Janković R. Preoperative preparation of patients with infectious and restrictive respiratory diseases as comorbidities. Acta Chir Iugosl. 2011;58(2):63–9.

Chapter 33
Chronic Kidney Disease

Sabeena Setia

BACKGROUND

Chronic kidney disease (CKD) affects approximately 1 in 10 of American adults and its incidence is increasing [1, 2]. Patients with CKD are at increased risk of perioperative morbidity and mortality even when adjusting for comorbid conditions such as hypertension and diabetes [3]. Newer data show that even patients with mild to moderate renal disease undergoing intermediate risk orthopedic and general surgery have higher rates of morbidity and increased length of hospital stay [4, 5]. Nonetheless, patients with CKD can safely undergo surgery with appropriate medical management.

PREOPERATIVE EVALUATION

The major morbidity and mortality in patients with end-stage renal disease (ESRD) is cardiovascular disease.
- Largest single cause of death is arrhythmias [6].
- Incidence of left ventricular hypertrophy is as high as 30 % in patients with CKD not yet on dialysis.
- Incidence of pulmonary hypertension in patients with ESRD may be as high as 40 % [6].

Given these comorbidities, a thorough preoperative cardiovascular and pulmonary risk assessment is crucial.
- Document history of existing renal disease, including etiology, onset, severity (e.g., CKD stage), and history of transplant
- Obtain baseline creatinine and electrolytes

M.B. Jackson et al. (eds.), *The Perioperative Medicine Consult Handbook*, DOI 10.1007/978-3-319-09366-6_33,
© Springer International Publishing Switzerland 2015

- Document history of renal problems in the past (e.g., history of contrast nephropathy)
- Screen patients at high risk of CKD by obtaining baseline creatinine and electrolytes

CKD affects renal drug elimination, drug absorption, drug distribution, and nonrenal clearance [7]. The normal creatinine clearance (CrCl) is generally >100 mL/min. Patients need adjustments to most commonly used medications when the CrCl falls below 50 mL/min. Glomerular filtration rate and/or CrCl is estimated using the Modification of Diet in Renal Disease (MDRD) study or using Cockcroft–Gault equation. These estimates are less accurate in certain circumstances, including when patients have more or less muscle mass [8].

Care for patients with hemodialysis-dependent ESRD or history of renal transplant should be coordinated with a nephrologist. Obtain the following information preoperatively:

- History of vascular access (anatomic location, history of clotting or stenosis).
- The patient's usual dialysis days and length of time is helpful information in coordinating hemodialysis care—it is preferable that hemodialysis (HD) is carried out on the day before surgery to minimize any risks from anticoagulation and from unresolved fluid or electrolyte shifts [8].
- The patient's "dry weight" prior to surgery, to guide management of volume status.

PERIOPERATIVE MANAGEMENT

CONTRAST-INDUCED NEPHROPATHY

Patients with CKD are at increased risk for contrast-induced kidney injury. Prospective data and meta-analysis on the use of oral N-acetylcysteine (NAC) have yielded conflicting results [9] though most practitioners would agree that it does not pose significant risk to the patient and is not excessively costly. IV hydration both before and after contrast is likely beneficial, though the jury is out as to whether isotonic sodium bicarbonate or isotonic normal saline is the preferred IV fluid [10].

When a Study or Procedure Requiring Contrast Is Proposed

1. Consider the necessity of the procedure and any alternatives (ultrasound, non-contrast CT scan, or MRI without gadolinium).

2. Iso-osmolar or low-osmolar iodinated contrast agents are preferred over high-osmolar iodinated contrast. Discuss options with radiologist.
3. If the test is required, pre-hydrate with IV fluids and consider the use of N-acetylcysteine prior to contrast procedure [9]:
   - If using sodium bicarbonate, administer a bolus of 3 mg/kg of isotonic bicarbonate for 1 h prior to the procedure and continue at a rate of 1 mL/kg/h for 6 h after the procedure.
   - If using normal saline, begin 1 mL/kg per hour at least 2 and preferably 6-12 h prior to the procedure, and continue for 6–12 h after contrast administration. The duration of administration of fluid should be directly proportional to the degree of renal impairment.
   - N-Acetylcysteine, at a dose of 1,200 mg orally twice daily, should be administered the day before and on the day of the procedure (Note: Protocols vary between 600 and 1,200 mg twice daily).

FLUID AND ELECTROLYTES

Patients who are above their dry weight are at risk of pulmonary edema and poorly controlled hypertension, while those who are under their dry weight are at risk of hypotension in the postoperative setting. Common electrolyte disturbances include hyperkalemia and metabolic acidosis—monitor and treat in the pre- and postoperative setting to reduce the risk of ventricular arrhythmia.

MEDICATIONS

It is crucial to review the pre-op medication list looking for drugs that may impair renal function or which require dose adjustment according to the patient's estimated CrCl.

- ACE-I and ARBs should generally be held on the morning of surgery (see Chap. 4).
- Useful resources include Micromedex®, e-books, and textbooks such as the ACP guide for renal dosing [11].
- Clinical pharmacists are helpful resources for dose adjustment recommendations.
- Nephrotoxic antibiotics (vancomycin, aminoglycosides, etc.) not only need dose adjustment but also close monitoring in the inpatient setting.
- Avoid nonsteroidal anti-inflammatory agents (NSAIDs).
- Morphine and meperidine have metabolites that can accumulate with renal insufficiency. Hydromorphone and fentanyl are the preferred narcotic agents for patient with renal insufficiency.

- Enoxaparin clearance is impaired by renal insufficiency—use with caution in patients with CKD (dose adjustments are available but close monitoring of anti-factor Xa is recommended).
- Use caution reinstituting ACE inhibitors and ARBs—monitoring renal function and electrolytes closely in the postoperative period.

ANEMIA AND COAGULOPATHY

Loss of erythropoietin production as renal function declines often leads to significant anemia. There has been vigorous debate in the literature as to defining the appropriate and safe target hemoglobin for patients with CKD. In general, erythropoietin-stimulating agents (ESAs) and supplemental iron (PO/IV) are used to maintain an Hgb concentration between 10 and 11.5 % and no higher than 13 % [12]. In the preoperative period, discussion with nephrology can be helpful in optimizing anemia prior to surgery with the knowledge that benefit of ESAs and supplemental iron takes a number of weeks to achieve.

Patients with CKD and ESRD demonstrate varying defects in hemostasis ranging from pro-thrombotic effects to dysfunctional platelets. As CKD progresses, pro-coagulopathic effects persist; however, platelet dysfunction increases risk of perioperative cutaneous, mucosal, and serosal bleeding [13]. The risk of uremic bleeding can be reduced by hemodialysis, desmopressin, cryoprecipitate, estrogen, or transfusion. Such strategies are best carried out in consultation with a nephrologist or hematologist.

REFERENCES

1. Kalamas AG, Neimann CU. Patients with chronic kidney disease. Med Clin North Am. 2013;97(6):1109–122.
2. Centers for Disease Control and Prevention (CDC). Prevalence of chronic kidney disease and associated risk factors–United States, 1999–2004. MMWR Morb Mortal Wkly Rep. 2007;56(8):161–5.
3. Mathew A, Devereaux PJ, O'Hare A, et al. Chronic kidney disease and postoperative mortality: a systematic review and meta-analysis. Kidney Int. 2008;73:1069–81.
4. Ackland GL, Moran N, et al. Chronic kidney disease and postoperative morbidity after elective orthopedic surgery. Anesthes Analg. 2011;112(6):1375–81.
5. Gaber AO, Moore LW, et al. Cross-sectional and case-control analysis of the association of kidney function staging with adverse postoperative outcomes in general and vascular Surgery. Ann Surg. 2013;258(1):169–77.
6. Rainor D, Borthwick E, Ferguson A. Perioperative management of the hemodialysis patient. Semin Dial. 2011;24(3):314–26.
7. Krishnan M. Preoperative care of patients with kidney disease. Am Fam Physician. 2002; 66(8):1472–6.
8. Stevens LA, Coresh J, Greene T, Levey AS. Assessing kidney function—measured and estimated glomerular filtration rate. N Engl J Med. 2006;354:2473–83.

9. Rudnick MR. Prevention of radiocontrast media-induced acute kidney injury. UpToDate. 2013. http://www.uptodateonline.com. Accessed Jan 2014.
10. KDIGO Clinical practice guideline for acute kidney injury. Kidney Int Suppl. 2012; 2:8
11. Aronoff GR, Bennett WM, Berns JS, Brier ME, Kasbekar N, Mueller BA, Pasko DA, Smoyer WE. Drug prescribing in renal failure. 5th ed. ACP Press: Philadelphia, PA; 2007.
12. Berns JS. Anemia of chronic kidney disease: target hemoglobin/hematocrit for patients treated with erythropoietic agents. UpToDate. 2013. http://www.uptodateonline.com. Accessed Jan 2013.
13. Jalal DI, Chonchol M, Targher G. Disorders of hemostasis associated with chronic kidney disease. Semin Thromb Hemost. 2010;36(1):34–40.

Chapter 34
Acute Kidney Injury

Somnath Mookherjee and Joana Lima Ferreira

BACKGROUND

Acute kidney injury (AKI) is a common postoperative complication. The incidence of AKI after surgery may be as high as 36 % depending on the definition of kidney injury used, the length of time the patient is followed postoperatively, and the type of surgery [1]. Up to 7 % of these patients may go on to require renal replacement therapy (RRT) [2]. Some types of surgeries increase the risk of AKI [3]. The development of postoperative AKI is associated with an increased risk of 30-day readmission [4], length of stay [5, 6], and mortality [1, 5–7]. Therefore, it is important for the internal medicine consultant to consider the risk of postoperative renal failure and how it may be mitigated.

PREOPERATIVE EVALUATION

It is difficult to predict who will develop postoperative AKI. A general surgery acute kidney injury risk index has been described [8], but it is not in wide usage, perhaps because it is not evident what specific measures may reduce risk. Nevertheless, it is useful for the medicine consultant to identify high-risk patients by considering patient- and surgery-specific risk factors.

PATIENT-SPECIFIC RISKS
A large number of risk factors have been associated with the development of postoperative AKI. Patients with preexisting comorbidities tend to be at highest risk. Commonly reported risk factors derived

M.B. Jackson et al. (eds.), *The Perioperative Medicine Consult Handbook*, DOI 10.1007/978-3-319-09366-6_34,
© Springer International Publishing Switzerland 2015

from multivariate analyses from various patient populations and types of surgeries include:

- Lab abnormalities: anemia [9], hypoalbuminemia [6]
- Chronic medical problems: chronic kidney disease, congestive heart failure [8, 10], diabetes [8], ischemic heart disease [10], chronic obstructive pulmonary disease [6], peripheral vascular disease [11]
- Physical examination findings/patient characteristics: obesity [12], advanced age [8, 10, 13], male gender [6, 8], presence of ascites [8], hypertension [6, 8, 14]

SURGERY-SPECIFIC RISKS

In any type of surgery, intrarenal vascular tone can be disrupted due to fluid loss and/or systemic inflammatory response (SIRS) leading to renal ischemia and injury [2]. The following types of surgeries have been particularly associated with a higher risk of developing postoperative AKI:

- Cardiac surgery, especially if requiring cardiopulmonary bypass (CPB)
- Vascular surgery, especially if requiring cross-clamping or contrast
- Renal or urological surgeries
- Intraperitoneal surgery
- Emergency surgery

PERIOPERATIVE MANAGEMENT

DEFINITION OF ACUTE KIDNEY INJURY

Even small changes in serum creatinine (SCr) or transient decreases in urine output (UO) can be harbingers of renal failure and loss of function. Based on the RIFLE (risk, injury, failure, loss, end-stage disease) classification of diminished renal function as defined by the Acute Dialysis Quality Initiative (ADQI) Group [15], the Acute Kidney Injury Network (AKIN) provides a classification schema for AKI that is useful to consider when evaluating patients in the postoperative setting [16]:

- Stage 1: Increase in $SCr \geq 0.3$ mg/dL or ≥ 1.5–2-fold increase from baseline or UO < 0.5 mL/kg/h for >6 h
- Stage 2: Increase in $SCr \geq 2$–3-fold increase from baseline or UO < 0.5 mL/kg/h for >12 h
- Stage 3: Increase in $SCr \geq 3$-fold increase from baseline or $SCr \geq 4$ mg/dL with acute increase ≥ 0.5 mg/dL or UO < 0.3 mL/kg/h for >12 h or anuria for 12 h

PREVENTION OF POSTOPERATIVE KIDNEY INJURY

A recent Cochrane review did not find any pharmacologic intervention (including dopamine, diuretics, calcium channel blockers, angiotensin-converting enzyme [ACE] inhibitors, *N*-acetylcysteine, sodium bicarbonate, antioxidants, erythropoietin, or selected hydration fluids) that could reliably prevent the development of renal failure in patients with or without preexisting renal failure [17]. Statins may decrease the risk of postoperative AKI but further research is needed before widespread implementation. The majority of cases of AKI are probably largely unavoidable. Nevertheless, attention to key principles may decrease the risk of postoperative AKI:

- Maintain euvolemia based on ongoing clinical assessment— predetermined intravenous fluid rates may overshoot or undershoot actual fluid requirements.
- Maintain cardiac output—overexpansion of intravascular volume in patients with even mild cardiomyopathy or unrecognized myocardial infarction may be manifested as AKI.
- Hypotension and hypovolemia can lead to acute tubular necrosis (ATN), a common cause of postoperative AKI.
- Avoid diuretics unless needed to treat intravascular hypervolemia.
- See Chap. 4 for recommendations regarding management of ACE inhibitors and ARBs. In general, we recommend holding ACE inhibitors and ARBs the morning of surgery unless the patient is persistently hypertensive with a systolic blood pressure greater than 180. If the patient takes these medications in the evening, they may be held or decreased the evening prior to surgery.
- Anemia may be associated with the development of AKI—work up anemia (see Chap. 22) but note that blood transfusion has also been associated with AKI [6, 13].
- See Chap. 33 regarding the prevention of contrast-induced nephropathy.

EVALUATION OF POSTOPERATIVE ACUTE KIDNEY INJURY

Table 34.1 outlines some considerations of the etiology of AKI specific to the postoperative setting. The standard approach to AKI in the medical patient is applicable (e.g., considering pre-, intra-, and postrenal etiologies), but specific attention should be paid to the patient's additional perioperative risk factors. Important elements of the workup include:

- Review operative and anesthesia records: specifically assess for hypotension, blood transfusions, use of diuretics, use of contrast, use of CPB, length of cross-clamp time, urine output, and any operative complications.

TABLE 34.1 CONSIDERATIONS FOR THE ETIOLOGY OF POSTOPERATIVE AKI

Prerenal	Intrinsic renal	Postrenal
■ Hypotension after anesthesia induction ■ Insufficient intraoperative hydration ■ High nasogastric (NG) tube output ■ Increased vascular permeability ("third spacing") ■ Surgical site bleeding/drain output ■ Abdominal compartment syndrome ■ Gastrointestinal bleeding ■ Retroperitoneal bleeding	■ Acute tubular necrosis (ATN) related to intra- or postoperative hypotension ■ Rhabdomyolysis related to positioning/prolonged surgery ■ Embolism (or microemboli) with vascular surgery or CPB ■ Acute interstitial nephritis (AIN) related to antibiotics or diuretics ■ Contrast nephropathy ■ Prolonged cross-clamping in vascular surgery	■ Ureteral damage or compression ■ Bladder outlet obstruction/urinary retention

- Evaluate the patient for intravascular volume status (orthostatic vital signs, jugular venous pressure) and abdominopelvic surgical drain output (increased clear drain output that has a creatinine level greater than serum creatinine level may signify urinary leak).
- Review patient chart for recent contrast studies, ongoing and immediate postoperative urine output, surgical drain output, and nasogastric tube output.
- Urine analysis: muddy brown granular and epithelial cell casts suggest ATN; hematuria may suggest nephrolithiasis, ureteral trauma, or intrinsic renal insult; eosinophiluria may indicate interstitial nephritis; rhabdomyolysis is indicated by urine myoglobin without red blood cells in urinalysis.
- Urine labs: high urinary specific gravity, low urinary sodium, and <1 % fractional excretion of sodium (FENa) support the diagnosis of a prerenal etiology.

- Serum labs: CBC and metabolic panel.
- Studies to consider: bladder scan for post-void residual (perform in and out catheterization if bladder scan values are suspect), retroperitoneal ultrasound (US), or computed tomography (CT) scan (to assess for hydronephrosis, fluid collections).

PRINCIPLES OF MANAGEMENT

The treatment and further workup is predicated on the working diagnosis. Nephrology consultation may be required if establishing euvolemia or relieving urinary tract obstruction does not result in improvement. Of course, a nephrologist should be involved if renal replacement therapy is needed—for example, if the patient has acidosis, volume overload compromising organ function, significant hyperkalemia, or uremia. Key points in management include:

- For all patients, if urine output is difficult to quantify, place a urinary catheter – but remove this as soon as possible.
- In case of intravascular volume depletion, aggressive intravenous fluids (IVF) either with Lactated Ringers (LR) or normal saline (NS) with frequent clinical reassessment of volume status and UO.
- Volume overload and CHF: diurese in the usual fashion; work up for myocardial infarction if CHF is new for the patient.
- If there is obstruction which is not relieved by a urinary catheter, this usually merits rapid surgical or percutaneous intervention.

REFERENCES

1. Biteker M, et al. Incidence, risk factors, and outcomes of perioperative acute kidney injury in noncardiac and nonvascular surgery. Am J Surg. 2014;207(1):53–9.
2. Noor S, Usmani A. Postoperative renal failure. Clin Geriatr Med. 2008;24(4):721–9. ix.
3. Kumar AB, Suneja M. Cardiopulmonary bypass-associated acute kidney injury. Anesthesiology. 2011;114(4):964–70.
4. Brown JR, et al. Impact of perioperative acute kidney injury as a severity index for thirty-day readmission after cardiac surgery. Ann Thorac Surg. 2014;97(1):111–7.
5. Lopez-Delgado JC, et al. Influence of acute kidney injury on short- and long-term outcomes in patients undergoing cardiac surgery: risk factors and prognostic value of a modified RIFLE classification. Crit Care. 2013;17(6):R293.
6. Kim CS, et al. Incidence, predictive factors, and clinical outcomes of acute kidney injury after gastric surgery for gastric cancer. PLoS One. 2013;8(12):e82289.
7. Bihorac A, et al. Long-term risk of mortality and acute kidney injury during hospitalization after major surgery. Ann Surg. 2009;249(5):851–8.
8. Kheterpal S, et al. Development and validation of an acute kidney injury risk index for patients undergoing general surgery: results from a national data set. Anesthesiology. 2009;110(3):505–15.
9. Walsh M, et al. The association between perioperative hemoglobin and acute kidney injury in patients having noncardiac surgery. Anesth Analg. 2013;117(4):924–31.
10. Abelha FJ, et al. Determinants of postoperative acute kidney injury. Crit Care. 2009;13(3):R79.

11. Ishikawa S, Griesdale DE, Lohser J. Acute kidney injury after lung resection surgery: incidence and perioperative risk factors. Anesth Analg. 2012;114(6):1256–62.
12. Suneja M, Kumar AB. Obesity and perioperative acute kidney injury: A focused review. J Crit Care. 2014;29(4):694.e1–6.
13. Vellinga S, et al. Identification of modifiable risk factors for acute kidney injury after cardiac surgery. Neth J Med. 2012;70(10):450–4.
14. Naik BI, et al. Incidence and risk factors for acute kidney injury after spine surgery using the RIFLE classification. J Neurosurg Spine. 2014;20(5):505–11.
15. Bellomo R, et al. Acute renal failure – definition, outcome measures, animal models, fluid therapy and information technology needs: the Second International Consensus Conference of the Acute Dialysis Quality Initiative (ADQI) Group. Crit Care. 2004;8(4):R204–12.
16. Mehta RL, et al. Acute kidney injury network: report of an initiative to improve outcomes in acute kidney injury. Crit Care. 2007;11(2):R31.
17. Zacharias M, et al. Interventions for protecting renal function in the perioperative period. Cochrane Database Syst Rev. 2013;9, CD003590.

Chapter 35
Rheumatoid Arthritis

Elizabeth Kaplan

BACKGROUND

Patients with rheumatoid arthritis (RA) should receive the same preoperative cardiovascular, pulmonary, and other risk assessment as other patients. In addition, it is also important to specifically note how well patients' underlying rheumatologic disease is controlled, any comorbidities that may be related to their RA, and what rheumatologic medications they take. Certain RA patients may be at increased risk for perioperative complications because of systemic complications of their underlying disease, medication effects, cervical spine instability, and specific joint issues [1]. Coordinated care with the patient's rheumatologist is recommended.

PREOPERATIVE EVALUATION

GENERAL PRINCIPLES
- Evaluate the preoperative status of the patient's rheumatologic disease. In general, surgery during active flares of disease should be avoided.
- Assess for signs or symptoms of cardiac disease and pulmonary complications.
- Pay attention to specific joints that may be involved such as the cervical spine.
- Assess recent history of and current steroid use, including pulse of steroids within the last year, even if the patient is no longer taking steroids (see Chap. 14).
- Determine the level of immune suppression.

M.B. Jackson et al. (eds.), *The Perioperative Medicine Consult Handbook*, DOI 10.1007/978-3-319-09366-6_35, © Springer International Publishing Switzerland 2015

CARDIAC EVALUATION

Patients with RA are at increased risk of cardiovascular disease (particularly those with poorly controlled or long-standing RA disease) [2, 3]. RA is associated with a 59 % increase in the risk of cardiovascular death compared with the general population [4]. Cardiovascular risk stratification follows the same principles as with other patients (see current American College of Cardiology/American Heart Association algorithm and discussion, Chap. 6), keeping in mind the increased incidence of cardiovascular events in patients with RA compared to the general population [5]. In addition, it may be more difficult to assess risk because some RA patients have limited physical mobility [5].

PULMONARY COMPLICATIONS

Patients with RA may have a variety of pulmonary complications including fibrosis, bronchiolitis, and pleuritis. Depending on the severity, these conditions may impact the patient's pulmonary status in the perioperative period [2, 6]. Preoperative evaluation should include thorough history taking for signs/symptoms of these conditions and consideration of workup if the patient has undiagnosed pulmonary symptoms.

CERVICAL SPINE DISEASE

Underlying C1–C2 subluxation, atlantoaxial impaction, or subaxial disease can put patients at risk for cervical spine injury when a patient's neck is manipulated during surgery (for intubation or positioning) [7]. Consider cervical spine films flexion/extension if the patient has the following characteristics (which make the possibility of cervical spine disease more likely):

- Diagnosis of RA for >5 years
- Undergoing orthopedic surgery specifically for rheumatologic disease (suggests more severe overall rheumatologic disease)
- Any neurologic abnormality corresponding to the cervical spine on exam [2]

If plain films are abnormal or if the patient does have a neurologic abnormality, then a discussion with the patient's rheumatologist and anesthesiologist prior to the surgery is recommended in regard to obtaining an MRI of the cervical spine before surgery and/or if specific precautions for surgery should be taken

HISTORY AND PHYSICAL EXAM

Assess the following [2, 8]:

- Duration of disease (longer duration associated with more joint damage, particularly neck involvement).
- Current functional status.
- Specific joints affected.
- Current medications.
- Previous and current use of steroids.
- Extra-articular manifestations of disease.
- Previous complications associated with surgery.
- History of hoarseness, sore throat, and trouble with inspiration (may indicate cricoarytenoid arthritis). If cricoarytenoid arthritis is present, it may lead to difficulties with intubation or postoperative airway obstruction due to irritation from endotracheal tube) [2, 6].

WORKUP

Consider including the following testing [2]:

- CBC to look for leukopenia related to drugs, anemia related to drug-associated duodenal irritation, and/or bone marrow suppression.
- Liver function tests (LFTs) to assess for potential effects of some RA medications. Specifically, patients on methotrexate typically should have LFTS checked every 12 weeks if on stable dose, one month after dose increases, or more often if LFTs are abnormal.
- Renal function (also to assess for medication effects).
- Walking O2 sat, if history or suspicion of pulmonary complications of RA.
- Consider cervical films (as above).

PERIOPERATIVE MANAGEMENT

Postoperative management of the patient with RA should receive routine care with special attention to the following:

- Early mobilization and consideration of involvement of physical therapy
- Monitor for any signs of infection
- Watching the degree of anemia, especially if present preoperatively

- Attention to thromboembolism prophylaxis
- Medication management (discussed below) with specific attention to any interactions with new postoperative medications

MEDICATION MANAGEMENT

See Table 35.1 for specific recommendations. Note that dosing of medication should be confirmed with the patient's pharmacy and/or rheumatologist. Consider discussing medication management with the patient's rheumatologist and surgeon if there are any questions.

TABLE 35.1 PERIOPERATIVE MANAGEMENT OF ANTIRHEUMATIC AGENTS

Methotrexate	• Usually given once weekly • A prospective randomized trial of patients with RA undergoing elective orthopedic surgery showed fewer complications, infections, and flares in the group that continued methotrexate rather than discontinuing [2, 8] • A 2008 review of the eight studies of methotrexate in the orthopedic perioperative period suggested that the medication could be continued through surgery (with 6 of the 8 studies finding that methotrexate did not pose an infectious risk, while the other 2 did) [2]. No data in non-orthopedic surgery • Generally acceptable to continue, unless surgery is being done for a serious infection in which case it should be held [2]. Other reasons to consider stopping medication include postop infection, rising creatinine, prolonged NPO state, and patient over age 70 • Recommend discussing with the patient's rheumatologist
Leflunomide (Arava®)	• No clear data for the management of leflunomide, and discussion with the patient's rheumatologist is usually warranted • One trial showed no difference in wound healing in orthopedic surgery patients [9]; however, a second trial showed that it did affect wound healing • Consider stopping in patients in whom large wounds are anticipated • Note that long half-life (~2 weeks) may make complete discontinuation problematic

(continued)

TABLE 35.I (CONTINUED)

Sulfasalazine	■ Generally acceptable to continue [10]
Azathioprine	■ May be continued for minor procedures and held for a few days for major procedures, although no clear data to suggest that this is necessary [10]
Hydroxychloroquine (Plaquenil®)	■ Generally acceptable to continue ■ One retrospective study showed no difference in postoperative wound healing or infections [10]

TNF-alpha inhibitors— infliximab (Remicade®), adalimumab (Humira®), etanercept (Enbrel®), etc.	■ Some small studies ($n = 31$ or fewer) have not shown a difference in orthopedic surgery, but were likely underpowered [10–12]
	■ Until more studies can be done, general consensus is to hold these medications [10]
	■ We recommend discussion with the patient's rheumatologist and surgeon regarding the use of these agents in the perioperative period
	■ If decision is to hold the drug (which is most likely the case for moderate to higher risk procedures), hold based on ½ life and hold at least two half-lives. Half-lives are listed below:
	    Etanercept (Enbrel®): 3.5–5.5 days
	    Adalimumab (Humira®): 10–20 days
	    Infliximab (Remicade®): 9.5 days
	    Certolizumab (Cimzia®): 14 days
	    Golimumab (Simponi®): 14 days
	■ Postoperatively it is recommended to restart these agents once wound healing is complete and there is no evidence of infection; usually not earlier than 10–14 days postoperatively [10]

Janus-associated kinase (JAK) inhibitor: tofacitinib (Xeljanz®)	■ No studies available at this time with this specific drug although so far it is thought infectious risks are similar to TNF-alpha inhibitors ■ Discuss with the patient's rheumatologist
Anakinra (Kineret®), rituximab, abatacept (Orencia®)	■ Discuss with the patient's rheumatologist
NSAIDs	■ See Chap. 4, perioperative medication management

REFERENCES

1. Gardner G, Mandel B. Assessing and managing rheumatologic disorders. In: Jaffer A, Grant P, editors. Perioperative medicine: medical consultation and co-management. 1st ed. New Jersey: Wiley-Blackwell; 2012. p. 215–29.
2. Meune C, Touze E, Trinquart L, Alanore Y. Trends in cardiovascular mortality in patients with rheumatoid arthritis over 50 years: a systemic review and meta-analysis of cohort studies. Rheumatology (Oxford). 2009;48:1309.
3. Aviña-Zubieta JA, Choi HK, Sadatsafavi M, et al. Risk of cardiovascular mortality in patients with rheumatoid arthritis: a meta-analysis of observational studies. Arthritis Rheum. 2008;59:1690.
4. Shur P, Weyand C. Coronary artery disease in rheumatoid arthritis: Epidemiology, pathogenesis, and risk factors. In: UpToDate. Waltham, MA: Wolters Kluwer; 2012. http://www.uptodateonline.com. Last updated Oct 2012. Accessed Jan 2014.
5. Bissar L, Almoallim H, Alotaibi M, Alwafi S. Perioperative management of patients with rheumatic diseases. Open Rheumatol J. 2013;7:42–50.
6. Bandi V, Munnur U, Braman SS. Airway problems in patients with rheumatologic disorders. Crit Care Clin. 2002;18(4):749–65.
7. Kwek TK, Lew TW, Thoo FL. The role of perioperative cervical spine x-rays in rheumatoid arthritis. Anaesth Intensive Care. 1998;26:636.
8. Grennan DM, Gray J, Loudon J, et al. Methotrexate and early postoperative complications in patients with rheumatoid arthritis undergoing elective orthopaedic surgery. Ann Rheum Dis. 2001;60(3):214–7.
9. Tanaka N, Sakahashi H, Sato E, et al. Examination of the risk of continuous leflunomide treatment on the incidence of infectious complications after joint arthroplasty in patients with rheumatoid arthritis. J Clin Rheumatol. 2003;9:115–8.
10. Pieringer H, Stuby U, Biesenbach G. Patients with rheumatoid arthritis undergoing surgery: how should we deal with antirheumatic treatment? Semin Arthritis Rheum. 2007; 36(5):278–86.
11. Bibbo C, Goldberg JW. Infectious and healing complications after elective orthopaedic foot and ankle surgery during tumor necrosis factor-alpha inhibition therapy. Foot Ankle Int. 2004;25:331–5.
12. Giles JT, Bartlett SJ, Gelber AC, et al. Tumor necrosis factor inhibitor therapy and risk of serious postoperative orthopedic infection in rheumatoid arthritis. Arthritis Rheum. 2006;55:333–7.

Chapter 36
Systemic Lupus Erythematosus

Elizabeth Kaplan

BACKGROUND

Patients with systemic lupus erythematosus (SLE) have multisystem disease and thus an increased risk for multiple perioperative complications, including wound infection, renal insufficiency, cardiovascular events, and pulmonary embolus. There is a two- to sevenfold higher mortality rate for SLE patients undergoing both nonelective and elective hip and knee surgery compared to rheumatoid arthritis (RA) patients and controls independent of major medical comorbidities [1]. Additional studies have demonstrated that patients with SLE had a higher prevalence of preoperative coexisting medical conditions and postoperative major complications [2] as well as short-term perioperative outcomes [3].

PREOPERATIVE EVALUATION

CARDIAC EVALUATION
Patients with SLE have a higher risk for coronary artery disease (CAD) at a relatively younger age [4, 5]. Cardiovascular risk stratification follows the same principles as with other patients (see Chap. 6), keeping in mind the increased incidence of cardiovascular events in patients with SLE. In addition, the presence of antiphospholipid antibodies confers a risk for both heart valve disease as well as thrombosis [4, 6]. A murmur in a patient with antiphospholipid syndrome (APLS) may warrant a transthoracic echocardiogram especially if the murmur is grade 3 or greater or the patient has symptoms that may be related to valve dysfunction.

M.B. Jackson et al. (eds.), *The Perioperative Medicine Consult Handbook*, DOI 10.1007/978-3-319-09366-6_36,
© Springer International Publishing Switzerland 2015

HISTORY

Assess the following specifics about patients with SLE:

- Current functional status
- Cardiovascular disease history and current signs/symptoms of CAD or valvular heart disease
- History of thromboembolic disease (both arterial and venous)
- Presence of APLS, which may impact risk of bleeding and thromboembolic event
- Hematologic abnormalities
- Renal disease
- Presence of immune dysfunction
- History of Raynaud's syndrome
- Current medications, keeping in mind the risk of immunosuppression and risk of cytopenias
- Previous and current use of steroids

In addition, patients should be assessed for risk factors that may lead to worse perioperative outcomes including smoking, use of oral contraceptive pills (OCPs), blood pressure, and lipid control [4, 7].

PHYSICAL EXAM AND WORKUP

- Conduct a thorough physical exam with specific attention to cardiac exam (for murmurs) and for signs of active inflammatory disease (oral ulcers, inflammatory arthritis, facial rash, neurologic symptoms).
- Labs should be tailored to the specific anticipated surgical procedure; however, usually patients should have a recent complete blood count, coagulation profile, serum electrolyte levels, and renal function to establish any preexisting conditions (hematologic or renal) and to use for comparison if issues arise postoperatively [4, 8].

PERIOPERATIVE MANAGEMENT

GENERAL PRINCIPLES

- The presence of multisystem effects of SLE can lead to an increased risk of postoperative complications [8].
- Important perioperative issues are hematologic abnormalities, acute renal failure, immune dysfunction, thromboembolic disease, and possible cardiac events in the setting of underlying CAD [4].

- Postoperative fever in a lupus patient can have many possible etiologies; infection, thrombosis, and SLE flare should all be considered.
- In patients with established thromboembolic disease and APLS, bridging therapy for anticoagulation is recommended (see Chap. 18).
- In patients with Raynaud's phenomenon, hypothermia perioperatively should be limited to avoid digital ischemia.

MEDICATION MANAGEMENT

See Table 35.1 of this text for perioperative recommendations for commonly used inflammatory arthritis medications. Note that dosing of medications should be confirmed with the patient's pharmacy and/or rheumatologist. Keep in mind the risk of immunosuppression from medications balanced against the risk of a lupus flare if medications are held. Also consider whether a patient may be at risk for adrenal insufficiency if they have been on steroids long term.

REFERENCES

1. Domsic RT, Lingala B, Krishnan E. Systemic lupus erythematosus, rheumatoid arthritis, and postarthroplasty mortality: a cross-sectional analysis from the nationwide inpatient sample. J Rheumatol. 2010;37(7):1467–72.
2. Lin J, Chien-Chang L, Lee Y, Chih-Hsiung W, Huang W, Chen T. Adverse outcomes after major surgery in patients with systemic lupus erythematosus: a nationwide population-based study. Ann Rheum Dis 2014;73:9 1646–1651 Published Online First: 5 June 2013 doi:10.1136/annrheumdis-2012-202758
3. Yazdanyar A, Wasko MC, Scalzi LV, Kraemer KL, Ward MM. Short-term perioperative all-cause mortality and cardiovascular events in women with systemic lupus erythematosus. Arthritis Care Res (Hoboken). 2013;65(6):986–91.
4. Gardner G, Mandel B. Assessing and managing rheumatologic disorders. In: Jaffer A, Grant P, editors. Perioperative medicine: medical consultation and co-management. 1st ed. New Jersey: Wiley-Blackwell; 2012. p. 215–29.
5. Hak AE, Karlson EW, Feskanich D, Stampfer MJ, Costenbader KH. Systemic lupus erythematosus and the risk of cardiovascular disease: results from the nurses' health study. Arthritis Rheum. 2009;61(10):1396.
6. Zuily S, Regnault V, Selton-Suty C, Eschwège V, Bruntz JF, Bode-Dotto E, De Maistre E, Dotto P, Perret-Guillaume C, Lecompte T, Wahl D. Increased risk for heart valve disease associated with antiphospholipid antibodies in patients with systemic lupus erythematosus: meta-analysis of echocardiographic studies. Circulation. 2011;124(2):215.
7. Bissar L, Almoallim H, Albazli K, Alotaibi M, Alwafi S. Perioperative management of patients with rheumatic diseases. Open Rheumatol J. 2013;7:42–50.
8. Axelrod J, Shmerling R, Ramirez M. Preoperative evaluation and perioperative management of patients with rheumatic disease. Uptodate. Updated Oct 2012. Accessed Feb 2014.

Chapter 37
Gout and Pseudogout

Elizabeth Kaplan

BACKGROUND

Surgery is a risk factor for development of crystal arthropathy or for a flare of preexisting crystal arthropathy [1]. Gout or pseudogout should be considered in patients with joint pain, unexplained fever, leukocytosis, or difficulty with physical therapy. It is vital not to ignore the patient's joint exam, especially in patients who are slow to mobilize or who cannot give a history. Both gout and pseudogout are in the differential diagnosis of postoperative fever. Correctly diagnosing postoperative gout or pseudogout may lead to earlier treatment of the patient and help prevent barriers to postoperative recovery.

PREOPERATIVE EVALUATION

Assess for a history of gout, including frequency of flares, medication regimen (including frequency of steroid use), whether there were any previous postoperative gout attacks, and uric acid levels (if appropriate). Examine the patient for any signs of joint redness or swelling suggestive of an acute flare. If such signs are present, consider initiating workup and treat flare (if it is in fact a crystal arthropathy) prior to surgery.

M.B. Jackson et al. (eds.), *The Perioperative Medicine Consult Handbook*, DOI 10.1007/978-3-319-09366-6_37, © Springer International Publishing Switzerland 2015

PERIOPERATIVE MANAGEMENT

PREVENTION OF COMPLICATIONS

- Generally continue prophylactic medications (e.g., allopurinol) up until surgery and resume postoperatively when possible.
- Attention to adequate hydration.
- Be aware that some new medications may induce a gouty attack (e.g., diuretics, cyclosporine), especially in a susceptible patient with a history of gout.
- Mobilization is helpful.

MANAGEMENT OF COMPLICATIONS

Diagnosis

For an acute arthritis in the postoperative setting, consider the following:

- Location—crystal arthropathies are often in large joints (e.g., knee, ankle) and/or in joints that were previously involved in flares [2].
- Assess clinical suspicion for septic joint—arthrocentesis is often needed and indicated to rule out infection as well as to diagnose crystal disease [3].

Distinguishing Gout from Pseudogout

- Pseudogout is common. It can be important to distinguish from gout to avoid unnecessary uric acid-lowering therapy for the long term.
- Gout should be considered in patients with a history of gout, obesity, chronic kidney disease, or use of diuretics or calcineurin inhibitors. Flares tend to occur within 8 days after surgery [2]; however, they can occur up to 3 weeks postoperatively. Uric acid levels can vary in either direction (increased or decreased) at the time of an attack and should not be used to make or exclude the diagnosis.
- Pseudogout can also occur postoperatively. X-rays may show calcium pyrophosphate deposition, but this finding is neither specific nor sensitive for pseudogout.
- Arthrocentesis with examination of fluid for crystals remains the gold standard for diagnosis.

TREATMENT OF ACUTE POSTOPERATIVE GOUT OR PSEUDOGOUT

- Principles of management are generally the same for both syndromes.
- Typical medications used to treat acute crystal arthropathy may be relatively contraindicated in the immediate postoperative setting—always work with the surgery team to make the best treatment decision.
- Consider intra-articular injection, especially if flare is limited to one joint. This can be especially useful if the other typical oral medications cannot be used in the postoperative period.
- Nonsteroidal anti-inflammatory medications—may be contraindicated in renal failure or surgical bleeding risk [3].
- Prednisone—may be contraindicated for concerns of wound healing, hyperglycemia, and infection risk.
- Colchicine—GI side effects may limit the use in patients post-abdominal surgery.
- IL-1 inhibitor such as anakinra—expensive and may be contraindicated because of concerns about effects on wound healing. Recommend involving rheumatology service if this medication is considered.
- For difficult cases, consultation with a rheumatologist may be necessary.

REFERENCES

1. Craig MH, Poole GV, Hauser CJ. Postsurgical gout. Am Surg. 1995;61(1):56–9.
2. Kang EH, Lee EY, Lee YJ, Song YW, Lee EB. Clinical features and risk factors of postsurgical gout. Ann Rheum Dis. 2008;67(9):1271–5.
3. Gardner G, Mandel B. Assessing and managing rheumatologic disorders. In: Jaffer A, Grant P, editors. Perioperative medicine: medical consultation and co-management. 1st ed. New Jersey: Wiley-Blackwell; 2012. p. 222–3.

Chapter 38
Bariatric Surgery

Ronald Huang and Ashok Reddy

BACKGROUND

Bariatric surgery is an effective long-term treatment for weight reduction [1–7], improving obesity-related comorbidities [1–7], and decreasing mortality [8, 9]. The National Institutes of Health (NIH) has developed consensus guidelines on appropriate candidates for bariatric surgery: body mass index (BMI) >40 or BMI between 35 and 40 with a serious obesity-related health problems including hypertension, diabetes mellitus (DM), hyperlipidemia, obstructive sleep apnea (OSA), obesity-hypoventilation syndrome (OHS), gastroesophageal reflux disease (GERD), and debilitating arthritis; acceptable operative risk; and ability to make necessary lifestyle changes and participate in long-term follow-up [10]. There is increasing support and evidence that bariatric surgery should be an option for patients with BMI between 30 and 35 with comorbidities [11].

The most common bariatric surgeries performed are the Roux-en-Y gastric bypass (RYGB) (open and laparoscopic), laparoscopic adjustable gastric band (LAGB), and the laparoscopic sleeve gastrectomy (LSG). A description of the most common surgeries is shown in Table 38.1. The 30-day mortality rate is approximately 0.1 % for each of these bariatric surgeries [1, 3, 5–7].

PREOPERATIVE EVALUATION

- The purpose of the preoperative evaluation for bariatric surgery is to assess the risk of complications, to identify and optimize medical conditions that increase a patient's risk, and to

M.B. Jackson et al. (eds.), *The Perioperative Medicine Consult Handbook*, DOI 10.1007/978-3-319-09366-6_38,
© Springer International Publishing Switzerland 2015

TABLE 38.1 DIFFERENCES BETWEEN ROUX-EN-Y GASTRIC BYPASS, LAPAROSCOPIC ADJUSTABLE GASTRIC BAND, AND LAPARO-SCOPIC SLEEVE GASTRECTOMY

Surgery	Roux-en-Y gastric bypass (RYGB)	Laparoscopic adjustable gastric band (LAGB)	Laparoscopic sleeve gastrectomy (LSG)
Description	Involves making a small pouch of the stomach, just below the esophagus, that empties into a loop of jejunum. Surgery can be performed both open and laparoscopically	A device is placed around the uppermost portion of the stomach and can be adjusted to allow tailoring of the stoma outlet	The stomach is reduced in size by removal of a large portion of the stomach following the major curvature of the stomach
Images			
% Excess weight loss [7][a]			
1 year	63.31 %	34.26 %	51.49 %
5 years	64.92 %	57.23 %	-

Figures reprinted with permission, Cleveland Clinic Center for Medical Art & Photography © 2005–2012. All Rights Reserved

[a]% excess weight loss = (weight loss/excess weight) × 100, excess weight = preoperative weight-ideal weight

TABLE 38.2 OBESITY SURGERY MORTALITY RISK SCORE (OS-MRS) PRIOR TO BARIATRIC SURGERY [13]

Class based on OS-MRS (points)	Mortality (90-day) (%)
A (0–1)	0.2
B (2–3)	1.2
C (4–5)	2.4

A point is given for BMI ≥ 50 kg/m^2, male gender, hypertension, known risk factors for PE (previous thromboembolism, IVC filter, hypoventilation, pulmonary hypertension), age ≥ 45

confirm that the patient meets the recommended criteria for bariatric surgery [12].

- A validated 90-day mortality risk assessment tool for patients undergoing bariatric surgery is shown in Table 38.2 [13], but the data remains mixed [14]. A risk scoring system for serious complications is also available [15].
- Cardiac risk assessment and optimization is similar in obese patient as other patients undergoing noncardiac surgery (see Chap. 6), but can be challenging due to limitations of the cardiac evaluation and cardiac testing due to weight limits of myocardial perfusion scans and cardiac catheterization tables, technical limitations of echocardiogram, and poor functional capacity for exercise stress testing. A cardiologist should be consulted if there are questions in regard to appropriate noninvasive testing.
- Obesity-related comorbidities that influence preoperative cardiac assessment and management of obese patients include coronary artery disease (CAD), congestive heart failure (CHF), DM, chronic renal insufficiency, cerebrovascular disease, hypertension, and poor exercise capacity [16].
- Pulmonary risk assessment prior to bariatric surgery is important. Obese patients have increased demand for ventilation, increased work of breathing, respiratory muscle inefficiency, and decreased lung volumes. These conditions are made worse when the patient is supine, under anesthesia, and with insufflation during laparoscopy.
- Pulmonary conditions associated with obesity to explore in the preoperative period include OSA and OHS (see Chap. 29), pulmonary hypertension (see Chap. 30), cor pulmonale, and history of venous thromboembolic disease (see Chap. 31).

- Any testing by the preoperative medical consultant should be determined by the history and physical exam (e.g., consideration of echocardiogram in the setting of CHF, pulmonary hypertension, or poor exercise capacity suspected to be due to a cardiopulmonary cause).
- Bariatric surgeons often have their own protocols for preoperative testing. Depending on which type of bariatric surgery is planned, the preoperative evaluation may include ultrasound of the gallbladder, endoscopy, upper GI series, fasting blood work (CBC, CMP, lipid panel, HbA1c, TSH, vitamin D 25-OH, vitamin B12, iron studies, ferritin), ECG, CXR, PFTs (ABG, full spirometry, and lung volumes), or sleep study [12].
- Medications should be reviewed carefully in the preoperative setting to anticipate any necessary changes or possible complications following surgery. For those patients who are taking numerous medications, controlled or extended-release medications, or medications with narrow therapeutic indices, an evaluation by a pharmacist with experience in bariatric surgery patients should be considered.
- A dietician should meet with the patient to optimize the patient's nutrition prior to surgery and to prepare them for post-bariatric surgery diet. Many patients are placed on a very-low-calorie diet (1,000 cal per day for approximately 3 weeks) before surgery to significantly reduce liver volume and improve operative exposure of the stomach.
- Another important component to the preoperative evaluation is a psychosocial evaluation for substance abuse, psychiatric disease, or social circumstances that may hinder the patient's ability to make the necessary long-term lifestyle changes.

PERIOPERATIVE MANAGEMENT

NUTRITION
- Proper hydration and adequate nutrition are particularly important following bariatric surgery.
- Postoperative bariatric diets vary according to institution but most follow a similar progression. Patients are usually able to start a clear liquid diet within the first 24 h after surgery and advance to a full liquid or soft and pureed diet prior to discharge under the direction of an experienced dietician.

- Patients should be reminded to eat more slowly and to eat more frequent but smaller meals, to stop eating when they are full, and to separate food from fluids by at least 30 min.
- The dietary changes following bariatric surgery are typically better tolerated for patients undergoing LAGB as opposed to RYGB or LSG since the band is not tightened when it is placed initially.
- Bariatric patients are at risk for nutrient deficiencies. Following RYGB and LSG, patients are started on a multivitamin with minerals and iron per day, calcium 1,200–1,500 mg per day (calcium citrate is preferred as it does not require an acid environment for absorption), and vitamin D3 (cholecalciferol) 800–1,200 IU per day. Patients may require vitamin B12 supplementation following surgery.
- Following LAGB, patients are not at the same increased risk of nutrient deficiency as those who undergo RYGB or LSG, but these patients are typically given the same supplementation.

MEDICATION MANAGEMENT

- In the early postoperative period, most medications are crushed or given as a liquid. Controlled or extended-release medications cannot be crushed or changed into a liquid formulation, so they must be changed after surgery to immediate-release medications with more frequent dosing.
- Bariatric surgery changes the pharmacokinetics of many drugs. The increase in gastric pH and the decrease in intestinal surface area available for absorption can decrease the bioavailability of a medication. This is particularly important for medications with narrow therapeutic indices such as psychiatric, antiepileptic, or transplant medications. Drug levels can be checked for most of these medications and should be followed postoperatively.

Management of Diabetic Medications

- Diabetic patients are at risk for hypoglycemia postoperatively. Patients who undergo RYGB and LSG are at the greatest risk of hypoglycemia. In addition to decreased caloric intake and rapid weight loss after surgery, the anatomic changes following RYGB and LSG affect hormone signaling and glucose metabolism. These patients may have dramatic decreases in the amount of insulin that they require starting on the first day or two after surgery. Patients who undergo LAGB have comparatively slower improvements in glucose control.

- Regardless of the type of bariatric surgery, all patients with diabetes should have their blood glucose monitored frequently after surgery.
- Oral sulfonylureas (glipizide, glyburide, and glimepiride) and meglitinides (repaglinide, nateglinide) should be discontinued after bariatric surgery.
- Metformin should be held postoperatively but lower doses can safely be resumed once acceptable renal function is confirmed.
- Patients taking insulin preoperatively are initially managed postoperatively with an insulin infusion protocol while NPO (see Chap. 13). When transitioning to SC insulin, basal insulin requirements are usually significantly reduced. Basal insulin dosing following bariatric surgery varies from patient to patient, but a rough starting point is half of the patient's basal insulin dose prior to surgery, the same dose as if a patient were not eating.
- Due to the substantial decrease in calories during the postoperative period, patients must be careful with prandial and correctional insulin. Both prandial and correctional insulin are typically not recommended upon discharge. Further adjustments are made in the outpatient setting.

Management of Antihypertensive Medications
- Patients who are taking antihypertensives are at risk for hypotension, electrolyte abnormalities, and dehydration postoperatively.
- Antihypertensive medications should be resumed carefully after bariatric surgery. Although most patients will still require antihypertensive medications at discharge, they may be able to achieve adequate blood pressure control with reduced doses or fewer medications.
- Patients receiving preoperative beta-blockers for cardiovascular indications should have these continued postoperatively (see Chap. 8).
- Diuretic agents are typically discontinued after bariatric surgery but may need to be continued or decreased in patients with CHF.

EARLY POSTOPERATIVE COMPLICATIONS
Anastomotic Leaks
- Leaks are potentially fatal and are important to recognize. The rate of anastomotic leak for RYGB has been reported to be 0.6–0.8 %, and the rate for LSG has been reported to be 0.7–0.9 % [5, 6].

- Signs and symptoms include new or worsening abdominal complaints, sustained tachycardia, or respiratory distress. Anastomotic leaks can be evaluated with an upper gastrointestinal (UGI) study or by CT.
- If there is a high suspicion for a leak, exploratory surgery is indicated despite negative studies.

Venous Thromboembolism

- Pulmonary embolism (PE) is one of the most common causes of mortality following bariatric surgery. The rates of pulmonary embolism (PE) for RYGB, LSG, and LAGB have recently been reported as 0.2 %, 0.3 %, and 0.02 %, respectively [5].
- The presenting symptoms of PE can be similar to anastomotic leaks and both should be considered in the appropriate clinical context.
- Anticoagulation is indicated when there is a high suspicion for PE. Anticoagulation can usually be started safely within 24–48 h after surgery, but this must be discussed with the surgeon.
- There is no consensus about prophylactic VTE regimens, but patients should receive sequential compression devices in addition to heparin or low-molecular-weight heparin. Extended prophylaxis after discharge is commonly employed as the time period of increased risk of VTE extends beyond discharge [17]. The duration of extended prophylaxis varies from institution to institution from 10 days to 4 weeks. Patients should also be encouraged to ambulate early.

Respiratory Failure

- Respiratory failure is a significant cause of morbidity following bariatric surgery. The rates of respiratory failure for RYGB, LSG, and LAGB have recently been described to be 1.3 %, 0.8 %, and 0.3 %, respectively [6].
- The prevention and treatment of respiratory failure include aggressive pulmonary toilet, incentive spirometry, oxygen supplementation, and early use of continuous positive pressure ventilation (CPAP) or bi-level positive airway pressure (BPAP) postoperatively when indicated. Medications that result in respiratory depression should be avoided or minimized.

Cardiac Complications

- The rate of myocardial infarction or cardiac arrest is approximately 0.1 % [5, 6].

- The prevention and management of cardiac complications following bariatric surgery are the same as for other surgeries and include close monitoring in high-risk patients, perioperative beta-blockade if indicated (see Chap. 8), and blood pressure control.

Bleeding

- Bleeding occurs at a higher rate (1 %) in RYGB compared with LSG (0.6 %) and LAGB (0.05 %) [5]. Indications to transfuse blood products are the same as for other surgical procedures (see Chap. 22). Patients may require an operative intervention if bleeding is persistent or severe.

Wound Complications

- Wound complications range in severity and include superficial and deep infections and wound dehiscence. Definitions vary by study along with the rates of wound complication. Wound complications are more common in open RYGB than any other procedure [5]. Wound complications are primarily managed by the surgical team.

REFERENCES

1. Buchwald H, Avidor Y, Braunwald E, Jensen MD, Pories W, Fahrbach K, et al. Bariatric surgery: a systematic review and meta-analysis. JAMA. 2004;292:1724–37.
2. Sjöström L, Lindroos AK, Peltonen M, Swedish Obese Subjects Study Scientific Group, et al. Lifestyle, diabetes, and cardiovascular risk factors 10 years after bariatric surgery. N Engl J Med. 2004;351(26):2683–93.
3. Maggard MA, Shugarman LR, Suttorp M, et al. Meta-analysis: surgical treatment of obesity. Ann Intern Med. 2005;142(7):547–59.
4. Colquitt JL, Picot J, Loveman E, et al. Surgery for obesity. Cochrane Database Syst Rev. 2009;2, CD003641.
5. Hutter MM, Schirmer BD, Jones DB, et al. First Report from the American College of Surgeons Bariatric Surgery Center Network: laparoscopic sleeve gastrectomy has morbidity and effectiveness positioned between the band and the bypass. Ann Surg. 2011;254:410–22.
6. Carlin AM, Zeni TM, English WJ, Michigan Bariatric Surgery Collaborative, et al. The comparative effectiveness of sleeve gastrectomy, gastric bypass, and adjustable gastric banding procedures for the treatment of morbid obesity. Ann Surg. 2013;257(5):791–7.
7. Chang SH, Stoll CR, Song J, et al. The effectiveness and risks of bariatric surgery: an updated systematic review and meta-analysis, 2003–2012. JAMA Surg. 2013;149(3):275–87.
8. Sjöström L, Lindroos AK, Peltonen M, Swedish Obese Subjects Study Scientific Group, et al. Effects of bariatric surgery on mortality in Swedish obese subjects. N Engl J Med. 2007;357(8):741–52.
9. Adams TD, Gress RE, Smith SC, et al. Long-term mortality after gastric bypass surgery. N Engl J Med. 2007;357(8):753–61.
10. Consensus Development Conference Panel. NIH conference: gastrointestinal surgery for severe obesity. Ann Intern Med. 1991;115(12):956–61.
11. ASMBS Clinical Issues Committee. Bariatric surgery in class I obesity (body mass index 30-35 kg/m^2). Surg Obes Relat Dis. 2013;9(1):e1–10.

12. Mechanick JI, Youdim A, Jones DB, et al, American Association of Clinical Endocrinologists; Obesity Society; American Society for Metabolic & Bariatric Surgery. Clinical practice guidelines for the perioperative nutritional, metabolic, and nonsurgical support of the bariatric surgery patien--013 update: cosponsored by American Association of Clinical Endocrinologists, The Obesity Society, and American Society for Metabolic & Bariatric Surgery. Obesity (Silver Spring). 2013;21 Suppl 1:S1–27.
13. DeMaria E, Murr M, Byrne TK, et al. Validation of the obesity surgery mortality risk score in a multicenter study proves it stratifies mortality risk in patients undergoing gastric bypass for morbid obesity. Ann Surg. 2007;246(4):578–82.
14. Longitudinal Assessment of Bariatric Surgery (LABS) Consortium, Flum DR, Belle SH, King WC, et al. Perioperative safety in the longitudinal assessment of bariatric surgery. N Engl J Med. 2009;361(5):445–54.
15. Finks JF, Kole KL, Yenumula PR, Michigan Bariatric Surgery Collaborative, from the Center for Healthcare Outcomes and Policy, et al. Predicting risk for serious complications with bariatric surgery: results from the Michigan Bariatric Surgery Collaborative. Ann Surg. 2011;254(4):633–40.
16. Poiriere P, Alpert MA, Fleisher LA. Cardiovascular evaluation and management of severely obese patient undergoing surgery: a science advisory from the American Heart Association. Circulation. 2009;120:86–95.
17. Steele KE, Schweitzer MA, Prokopowicz G, et al. The long-term risk of venous thromboembolism following bariatric surgery. Obes Surg. 2011;21(9):1371–6.

Chapter 39
Decision-Making Capacity

Kara J. Mitchell

BACKGROUND

Surgeons obtain informed consent from patients for the procedures they perform. Occasionally, however, the medical consultant will be asked to assist with assessment of a particular patient's capacity (or lack thereof) to consent to evaluation and/or treatment. Patients are presumed to possess decision-making capacity, unless a clinical evaluation suggests that it is lacking [1–3]. Studies suggest, however, that clinicians frequently fail to recognize when patients lack decision-making capacity [1, 3].

Often, the decision-making capacity of patients is questioned only when:

- The decision to be made is particularly risky or complex, *or*
- The decision that a patient has made is in conflict with what a provider has recommended [2, 3].

RISK FACTORS FOR LOSS OF DECISION-MAKING CAPACITY

WHAT RISK FACTORS SUGGEST THAT A PATIENT MAY LACK MEDICAL DECISION-MAKING CAPACITY? [2, 3]

- Developmental delay
- Alzheimer disease and other forms of dementia or cognitive impairment
- Psychiatric illness
- Residence in a skilled nursing facility (SNF)
- Parkinson's disease

M.B. Jackson et al. (eds.), *The Perioperative Medicine Consult Handbook*, DOI 10.1007/978-3-319-09366-6_39, © Springer International Publishing Switzerland 2015

- Hospitalization for medical illness
- Diagnosis of brain tumor or traumatic brain injury

Note that a significant percentage of patients with these risk factors, including those with psychosis, dementia, or developmental delay, will possess decision-making capacity.

DO PATIENTS WITH DEMENTIA ALWAYS LACK DECISION-MAKING CAPACITY?

No. Measures of cognitive function such as the mini-mental status examination (MMSE) correlate with decision-making capacity at high scores (indicating that the patient is more likely to have capacity) and low scores (indicating that the patient is less likely to have capacity); however, patients with low scores may still possess decision-making capacity, and patients with high scores may lack it. MMSE scores between 20 and 24 have no effect on the likelihood that the patient has decision-making capacity [1, 3, 4].

ASSESSMENT AND MANAGEMENT

HOW DO I DETERMINE IF MY PATIENT HAS DECISION-MAKING CAPACITY? [1, 3]

The provider must determine if the patient demonstrates specific abilities:

- Ability to communicate a choice
- Ability to understand relevant information (risks/benefits/ alternatives) regarding a proposed test or a treatment
- Ability to appreciate the current situation and its consequences
- Ability to manipulate information rationally

It is important to understand that while patients must demonstrate the ability to reason and communicate in order to make their own medical decisions, they are *not* required to make what the healthcare provider considers a "good" decision. In addition, take care to exclude the possibility of "pseudo-incapacity": the situation in which patients cannot understand information presented in medical jargon, nonnative language, rushed manner, or other improper format [3, 5].

- Speak in plain language
- Use hearing aids or other assistive devices when necessary
- Use proper translation
- Use diagrams and other communication tools
- Provide the opportunity to ask questions for clarification

WHAT TOOLS ARE AVAILABLE TO HELP ASSESS THE DECISION-MAKING CAPACITY OF PATIENTS?

The Aid to Capacity Evaluation is one of many available tools; this can be performed within 30 min, has been validated against a clinical gold standard, has a reasonable level of evidence to support its use, and is available online for free: http://www.jointcentreforbioethics.ca/tools/ace.shtml [3, 5]. Other advantages of this tool include the availability of free training materials, its focus on the actual decision to be made by your patient, and its facilitation of clinical documentation [2, 3, 5]. If the capacity assessment is complex, consider involving an appropriate specialty consultant or ethics committee [1–3].

CAN A PATIENT'S DECISION-MAKING CAPACITY CHANGE?

Yes. Decision-making capacity is influenced by time and situation [1–3]. For example, a patient may lack capacity while suffering from delirium, but regain full decision-making capacity when recovered from acute illness. Patients may also have limited decision-making capacity, depending upon the complexity of and the risks associated with the decision to be made. For example, a patient may have the capacity to make choices regarding diet, but lack capacity to elect major surgery with the attendant morbidity and mortality risks.

WHAT SHOULD I DO IF MY PATIENT LACKS DECISION-MAKING CAPACITY?

If a patient is found to lack capacity, efforts should be made to identify and treat any reversible contributing causes [1–3]. Potentially thought-altering medications, such as opiates or benzodiazepines, should *not* be withheld for the purposes of obtaining consent, as long as they are being administered properly and for an appropriate indication; withholding them can be construed as coercive. Moreover, pain and anxiety can actually contribute to incapacity, if left untreated.

What to do if incapacity is established varies by state and typically involves identification of an appropriate surrogate decision-maker or a guardian. Advance directives from the patient, if applicable, should be executed. In case of true emergency (and no appropriate directive or surrogate is available), it is generally acceptable to provide the evaluation and/or treatment to which a "reasonable person" would have consented [1]. Note that in some areas, surrogate decision-makers cannot legally give consent for certain "high-stakes" treatments, such as sterilization, amputation, or electroconvulsive therapy; in these cases, a court order may be required.

REFERENCES

1. Applebaum PS. Assessment of patients' competence to consent to treatment. N Engl J Med. 2007;357:1834–40.
2. Etchells E, Sharpe G, Elliott C, Singer PA. Bioethics for clinicians: 3 Capacity. CMAJ. 1996; 155:657–61.
3. Sessums LL, Zembrzuska H, Jackson JL. Does this patient have medical decision-making capacity? JAMA. 2011;306:420–7.
4. Folstein MF, Folstein SE, McHugh PR. "Mini-mental state": a practical method for grading the cognitive state of patient for the clinician. J Psychiatr Res. 1975;12:189–98.
5. Community tools: Aid to capacity evaluation (ACE). University of Toronto Join Centre for Bioethics. http://www.jointcentreforbioethics.ca/tools/ace.shtml. Accessed 25 Jan 2014.

Chapter 40
Perioperative Care of Elderly Patients

Sabeena Setia and G. Alec Rooke

BACKGROUND

Aging is associated with a loss of physiologic reserve and a consequent increase in perioperative risk. Comorbidities and age strongly interact to increase the rate of perioperative complications with the effect of comorbidities becoming more pronounced with increasing age [1]. Despite major advances in surgical and anesthetic techniques and perioperative optimization, elderly patients continue to shoulder the burden of complications, longer hospital stays, and institutionalization after surgery.

PREOPERATIVE EVALUATION

The effect of aging is difficult to quantify, but the concept of frailty is useful in assessing surgical risk. Frailty refers to the state of diminished physiological reserve across multiple organ systems that leads to an overall increased vulnerability to stress [2]. Various tools have been developed ranging from single measures of function such as grip strength or timed up and go (TUG) (Table 40.1) to detailed comprehensive geriatric assessments that include measures of cognitive ability [3, 4]. The Fried criteria, focusing on functional assessment, have been validated for elderly surgical patients and may be useful [5]. In addition, a frailty score, developed by Robinson et al. that includes cognitive assessment, albumin, and walking speed, has been shown to be helpful in risk stratification (Table 40.2) [6].

M.B. Jackson et al. (eds.), *The Perioperative Medicine
Consult Handbook*, DOI 10.1007/978-3-319-09366-6_40,
© Springer International Publishing Switzerland 2015

TABLE 40.1 THE TIMED UP AND GO (TUG) TEST

Equipment needed: Timer and chair

Directions: Patients wear their regular footwear and can use a walking aid if needed

Begin by having the patient sit back in a standard armchair and identify a line 10 feet away on the floor

Instructions to the patient: When I say "go," I want you to:

1. Stand up from the chair
2. Walk to the line on the floor at your normal pace
3. Turn
4. Walk back to the chair at your normal pace
5. Sit down again

On the word "go" begin timing

Stop timing after patient has sat back down and record the time: _____ seconds

Interpretation: ≤10 s, fast

                11–14 s, intermediate

                ≥15 s, slow (associated with increased postoperative complications and increased 1-year mortality)

Adapted with permission by [4]

PREOPERATIVE HISTORY AND PHYSICAL EXAMINATION

In addition to the standard preoperative evaluation, attention should be given to the following issues:

- History of surgical or anesthetic complications
- Identifying patients with likely diastolic dysfunction from echocardiography or a history of "heart failure" after surgery
- Nutritional status—calculate body mass index (BMI) and document unintended weight loss > 10–15 % within 6 months (see Chap. 41)
- Functional capacity and performance status: consider quantification via the TUG if patient is mobile; document deficits in vision, hearing, or swallowing; document history of falls ("Have you fallen in the past year?") [7]
- Cognitive function: if suspicious of poor baseline cognitive function, perform Mini-Cog screen (Table 40.2) [7]
- Frailty: among patients with multiple chronic diseases, consider additional quantification of functional impairment using a frailty assessment tool such as the Fried criteria (Table 40.3)

TABLE 40.2 TOOLS TO MEASURE FRAILTY

Method of measuring frailty	Impact of frailty on surgical outcome	Surgical population studied	Authors
Grip strength	Increased postoperative complications and increased LOS	All ages Elective major abdominal surgery	Klidjian et al. [15]
Timed Up and Go	Increased postoperative complications and 1-year mortality	Elective colorectal and cardiac ≥65 years old	Robinson et al. [4]
7 frailty traits Timed get Up and Go ≥ 15 s Katz score ≤ 5 Mini-Cog ≤ 3 Charlson index ≥ 3 Hct < 35 % Albumin < 3.4 Falls score > 1	Increased postoperative complications, increased LOS, higher 30-day readmission rates	Elective colorectal or cardiac surgery	Robinson et al. [6]
Edmonton Frail Scale Cognition General health Functional independence Social support Medication use Nutrition Mood Continence Functional performance	Increased postoperative complications, prolonged LOS, increased institutionalization rate	≥70 years old Lower limb orthopedic surgery Spinal surgery Abdominal surgery Vascular surgery	Dasgupta et al. [16]
Fried criteria Weight loss Decreased grip strength (weakness) Exhaustion Low physical activity Slowed walking speed	Increased postoperative complications, prolonged LOS, new institutionalization at discharge	≥65 years old Elective surgery (major and minor)	Makary et al. [5]

Adapted with permission from Oxford University Press on behalf of the British Geriatrics Society [2]

TABLE 40.3 MINI-COG SCREEN: 3-ITEM RECALL AND CLOCK DRAW

1. Get the patient's attention and then say:

   "I am going to say three words that I want you to remember now and later. The words are:

   Banana   **Sunrise**   **Chair**

   Please say them for me now."

   Give the patient 3 tries to repeat the words. If unable after 3 tries, go to next item

2. Say all the following phrases in this order:

   "Please draw a clock in the space below. Start by drawing a large circle. Put all the numbers in the circle and set the hands to show 11:10 (10 past 11)."

   If the subject has not finished clock drawing in 3 min, discontinue and ask for recall items

3. Say: "What were those three words I asked you to remember?"
   Scoring:

3-item recall (0–3 points):	1 point for each correct word
Clock draw (0 or 2 points):	0 points for abnormal clock[a]

[a]A normal clock has all of the following elements: (a) All numbers 1–12, each only once, present in the correct order and direction inside the circle, (b) Two hands are present, one pointing to 11 and the other pointing to 12. Any clock missing any of these elements is scored abnormal. Refusal to draw a clock is scored abnormal

Interpretation of Mini-Cog [4]

Total score of 0, 1, or 2 suggests possible impairment

Total score of 3, 4, or 5 suggests no impairment

© Soo Borson MD [7], used with permission of the author

- Identifying alcohol and substance use: among patients 65 years or older, the prevalence of binge drinking is as high as 14.5 % among men and 3.3 % among women [8].
- Use of multiple psychoactive medications.

PREOPERATIVE LABS AND STUDIES

- Obtain hemoglobin in all patients >80 years of age, those undergoing operations in which significant blood loss is expected, or in patients who have symptoms suggestive of severe anemia.
- Obtain renal function tests in all elderly patients, especially those who are undergoing high-risk surgery, having diabetes and cardiovascular disease, or using ACE-I, diuretics, or NSAIDs.

- Consider serum albumin as a marker of frailty.
- See Chap. 6 for recommendations on preoperative electrocardiogram (ECG); consider in some patients over the age of 70, as finding a significant abnormality may influence risk assessment and will provide a baseline to help interpret changes postoperatively. Importantly, recognize that most elderly patients will have age-related ECG abnormalities that will not change perioperative management.

ORGAN SYSTEM SPECIFIC RISKS IN THE ELDERLY

The medicine consultant should anticipate problems and complications and help outline a plan to prevent them. Specific considerations include:

- Increased risk of both underlying coronary artery disease (CAD) and multivessel CAD; risk is greatest beyond 70 years of age.
- Decreased ability to tolerate either extreme of volume status.
- Increased risk of renal drug toxicity; glomerular filtration rate (GFR) is reduced by approximately 10 % per decade and should be assessed pre- and postoperatively in the elderly.
- Increased risk of delirium due to cognitive dysfunction, age, polypharmacy, poor nutrition, electrolyte abnormalities, hearing/vision impairment, depression, sleep deprivation, and comorbidities.
- Increased risk of pulmonary complications, due to small airway collapse from a loss of lung tissue elasticity, increased work of breathing due to increased chest stiffness and a barrel chest, and risk of aspiration from impaired swallowing and diminished airway protective reflexes.
- Higher risk of atelectasis, hypoxia, pneumonia, respiratory failure, prolonged ventilation, silent aspiration, and pneumonia (see Chap. 27).

At this point, the stress of the proposed surgery must be evaluated, especially if large fluid requirements are expected due to hemorrhage or third spacing. Time of recuperation is typically longer in older patients and could represent an unacceptably high percentage of expected remaining lifespan. Less stressful palliative procedures may need to be considered. Remember that the goals of surgery are often different for elderly patients, where there is greater concern over preservation of function and independence rather than mere prolongation of life.

PERIOPERATIVE MANAGEMENT

PREOPERATIVE MANAGEMENT

Once the decision is made to proceed with surgery, efforts should be made to prevent common complications in this age group. Although frailty indices may help to identify patients at higher risk, the challenge lies in whether this risk can be modified. Comprehensive geriatric assessments (CGA) and multidisciplinary geriatric interventions implemented preoperatively have been shown to reduce complications, including delirium, pneumonia, delayed mobilization, and length of stay in various surgical populations including oncology, orthopedic, and cardiothoracic patients [9–11].

Preoperative exercise programs ("prehabilitation") with the goal of improving strength and functional ability have also shown some benefit but need further study [12, 13]. These interventions require a comprehensive coordinated care team, including geriatricians, physical therapists, and social workers—the medicine consultant should explore what resources are available at their institutions. At a minimum, the medicine consultant should coordinate with the patient's primary care provider to discontinue nonessential medications preoperatively and prepare the patient and family for the likely postoperative rehabilitation course. Frank and open communication with the surgery team regarding the appropriateness of alternate procedures, surgery-specific risks, and expected recovery time is essential in anticipating complications. The medical consultant, the primary care physician, and the surgeon should ideally be in consensus about the necessity, expected risks, and outcomes of the proposed procedure.

POSTOPERATIVE MANAGEMENT
Minimize the Risk of Delirium (see Chap. 46)
- Avoid anticholinergics and antihistamines
- Benzodiazepines, narcotics, and sleep agents should be administered with caution
- Minimize polypharmacy in general—see updated Beers criteria for medications that should be avoided [14]
- Ensure adequate quiet during sleep hours
- Frequent reminders for orientation

Optimize Pain Management
Postoperative pain increases the risk of adverse outcomes in elderly patients by contributing to cardiac ischemia, tachycardia, hypertension, hypoxemia, and delirium. Pain is often undertreated in the

elderly out of concern for risks associated with opiates, including delirium and constipation. In conjunction with pain management services, the medicine consultant should make specific recommendations regarding analgesia:

- Avoid meperidine
- Consider adjunctive therapies such as acetaminophen, gabapentin, lidocaine or capsaicin patches, and local anesthesia or regional anesthesia
- Avoid NSAIDs in most cases

Other Measures Likely to Be Salutary in the Elderly

- Aggressive pulmonary toilet and aspiration precautions to prevent pulmonary complications
- Aggressive prevention and treatment of constipation with routine stool softeners and encouraging oral hydration when possible
- Frequent checks for signs of pulmonary congestion, especially on post-op day 2 or 3 when third space fluid is mobilized
- Minimize the introduction of new medications to decrease risk of polypharmacy
- Follow renal function

REFERENCES

1. Tiret L, Desmonts JM, Hatton F, et al. Complications associated with anaesthesia: a prospective survey in France. Can Anesth Soc J. 1986;33:336.
2. Partridge JSL, Harari D, Dhesi JK. Frailty in the older surgical patient: a review. Age Ageing. 2012;41:142–47.
3. Mathias S, Nayak USL, Isaacs B. Balance in elderly patients: the "get-up and go" test. Arch Phys Med Rehabil. 1986;67:387–9.
4. Robinson TN, Wu DS, Sauaia A, et al. Slower walking speed forecasts increased postoperative morbidity and one-year mortality across surgical specialties. Ann Surg. 2013;258(4):582–90. doi:10.1097/SLA.0b013e3182a4e96c.
5. Makary MA, Segev DL. Frailty as a predictor of surgical outcomes in older patients. J Am Coll Surg. 2010;210(6):901–9089.
6. Robinson TN, Wu DS, Pointer M, Dunn CL, Cleveland Jr JC, Moss M. Simple frailty score predicts post-operative complications across surgical specialties. Am J Surg. 2013;206(4):544–50.
7. ACS NSQIP/AGS Best Practice Guidelines: optimal preoperative assessment of the geriatric surgical patient. http://site.acsnsqip.org/wp-content/uploads/2011/12/ACS-NSQIP-AGS-Geriatric-2012-Guidelines.pdf
8. Blazer DG, Wu LT. The epidemiology of substance use and disorders among middle aged and elderly community adults: National survey on drug use and health. Am J Psychiatry. 2009;166(10):1162–9.
9. Dewan SK, Zheng SB, Xia SJ. Preoperative geriatric assessment: comprehensive, multidisciplinary and proactive. Eur J Intern Med. 2012;23(6):487–94.
10. Harari D, Hopper A, Dhesia J, Babic-Illman G, Lockwood L, Martin F. Proactive care of older people undergoing surgery ("POPS"): designing, embedding, evaluating and funding a comprehensive geriatric assessment service for older elective surgical patient. Age Ageing. 2007;36:190–6.

11. Cheema FN, Abraham NS, Berger DH, Albo D, Taffet GE, Naik AD. Novel approaches to perioperative assessment and intervention may improve long-term outcomes after colorectal cancer resection in older adults. Ann Surg. 2011;253(5):867–74.

12. Mayo NE, Feldman L, Scott S, Zavorsky G, Kim do J, Charlebois P, Stein B, Carli F. Impact of preoperative change in physical function on postoperative recovery: argument supporting prehabilitation for colorectal surgery. Surgery. 2011;150(3):505–14. doi:10.1016/j.surg.2011.07.045.

13. Valkenet K, Van de Port IG, Dronkers JJ, deVries WR, Lindeman E, Backx FJ. The effects of preoperative exercise therapy on post-operative outcome: a systematic review. Clin Rehabil. 2011;25(2):99–111. doi:10.1177/0269215510380830.

14. American Geriatrics Society 2012 Beers Criteria Update Expert Panel. American Geriatrics Society updated Beers Criteria for potentially inappropriate medication use in older adults. J Am Geriatr Soc. 2012;60(4):616–31. doi:10.1111/j.1532-5415.2012.03923.x.

15. Klidjian AM, Foster KJ, Kammerling RM, Cooper A, Karran SJ. Relation of anthropometric and dynamometric variables to serious postoperative complications. Br Med J. 1980;281:899–901.

16. Dasgupta M, Rolfson DB, Stolee P, Borrie MJ, Speechley M. Frailty is associated with post-operative complications in older adults with medical problems. Arch Gerontol Geriatr. 2009;48:78–83.

Chapter 41
Nutrition

Tara Spector and Lindsay Frank

BACKGROUND

Nutrition assessment should be a routine part of any preoperative evaluation. Malnutrition is associated with increased rates of postoperative infection, impaired wound healing [1], and increased length of stay [2]. The stress of surgery causes catecholamine and cortisol release, which results in a hypermetabolic state that can further exacerbate underlying malnutrition [3]. Identifying patients with malnutrition and stratifying them according to severity of malnutrition allows for perioperative interventions that reduce surgical complications. In select cases, it may be beneficial to delay surgery for 5 to 7 days to optimize nutritional status to bolster the immune system and prepare the body for the systemic stress response to surgery.

In the perioperative and postoperative period, both well-nourished and malnourished patients benefit from interventions focused on optimizing nutritional state, including immunonutrition and minimization of time spent nil per os (NPO). Additionally, the consulting internist should be aware of recommendations regarding initiation of nutrition postoperatively, with a focus on early advancement of diet or enteral feeding.

PREOPERATIVE EVALUATION

EVALUATION OF NUTRITION STATUS
While there are no universally accepted criteria, most experts require two of the following to diagnose malnutrition: inadequate caloric intake, unintentional weight loss, low BMI, visible loss of muscle mass or subcutaneous fat, or poor handgrip strength [4]. Note that

M.B. Jackson et al. (eds.), *The Perioperative Medicine Consult Handbook*, DOI 10.1007/978-3-319-09366-6_41,
© Springer International Publishing Switzerland 2015

serum hepatic proteins such as the negative acute phase proteins albumin and prealbumin are NOT valid indicators of nutritional status, rather they more accurately reflect severity of disease/inflammation [5]. Furthermore, low levels of these serum proteins are not responsive to nutrition intake during an active inflammatory state [4]. A routine preoperative evaluation for nutritional status should include the following:

- History of recent weight loss and adequacy of caloric intake
- Identification of comorbid conditions that can influence nutritional status (i.e., prior GI surgery, chronic kidney disease, cancer, recent trauma, or infection)
- Identification of disease states that necessitate dietary restriction (e.g., congestive heart failure)
- Identification of significant alcohol or substance abuse history
- Physical exam: height, weight (to allow body mass index calculation), evidence of muscle wasting, ascites/edema
- Laboratory evaluation: if there is concern for malnutrition based on history and physical exam, order basic metabolic panel and phosphate level to evaluate for electrolyte abnormalities and renal dysfunction and a CBC to evaluate for anemia

RISK STRATIFICATION
Preoperative nutrition evaluation addresses both current nutritional status as well as the risk for nutritional deterioration as a result of increased demands caused by metabolic stress [5]. The Nutritional Risk Screening 2002 (NRS 2002) is a validated method for identifying malnourished patients that may benefit from nutritional support [5]. This tool also helps to classify patients with mild, moderate, or severe malnutrition. Details of this screening tool are found in Tables 41.1 and 41.2.

PERIOPERATIVE MANAGEMENT

OPTIMIZING NUTRITION STATUS PRIOR TO SURGERY
Preoperative Enteral and Parenteral Nutrition
Patients with severe malnutrition (defined as nutritional risk screen [NRS] greater than three or weight loss of 10–15 % of total body mass in the past six months or BMI <18.5) undergoing major elective surgery (i.e., gastrointestinal surgery, cardiothoracic surgery, complex head and neck surgery) benefit from supplemental nutrition prior to

TABLE 41.1 NUTRITIONAL RISK SCREENING (NRS 2002): INITIAL SCREENING [5]

	Yes	No
Is BMI < 20.5?		
Has the patient lost weight within the last 3 months?		
Has the patient had a reduced dietary intake in the last week?		
Is the patient severely ill? (e.g., in intensive therapy)		

Yes: If the answer is "Yes" to any question, the screening in Table 41.2 is performed
No: If the answer is "No" to all questions, the patient is rescreened at weekly intervals. If the patient is scheduled for a major operation, a preventative nutritional care plan is considered to avoid the associated risk status

surgery [6]. Just 5 to 7 days of adequate preoperative nutrition can prepare the body for the metabolic insult and stress of surgery and results in improved surgical outcomes including reduced rates of infection and surgical complications [7].

- Enteral nutrition is preferred to parenteral nutrition as it has lower risk of infection, is less expensive, and maintains the integrity of the gut mucosal lining. Supplemental nutrition (as oral supplements or by tube feeds) should provide 25 kcal/kg/day of calories and 1.5–2 g/kg/day of protein [7].
- If enteral nutrition is contraindicated (bowel obstruction, bowel ischemia, acute peritonitis) and the patient is severely malnourished, surgery should be delayed for 5 to 7 days to administer parenteral nutrition, if feasible.
- Parenteral nutrition should be stopped 2–3 h prior to surgery and then resumed the morning after surgery [8].

Immunonutrition
Immunonutrition formulas, or immune-modulating diets, are enteral feeding formulas that contain specific amino acids, vitamins, and minerals that become conditionally essential in periods of illness and stress [9]. Supplementation with these nutrients prior to and after surgery helps to enhance immune function and modulate the inflammation created by surgery. Several pharmaceutical companies produce these immune-modulating beverages, which are available online and through select pharmacies. While the use of immune-modulating

TABLE 41.2 NRS 2002: FINAL SCREENING [5]

Impaired nutritional status		Severity of disease (≈increase in requirements)	
Absent **Score 0**	Normal nutrition status	Absent **Score 0**	Normal nutritional requirements
Mild **Score 1**	Wt loss > 5 % in 3 months or food intake below 50–70 % of normal requirement in preceding week	Mild **Score 1**	Hip fracture; chronic patients with acute complications; cirrhosis; COPD; chronic hemodialysis; diabetes, oncology
Moderate **Score 2**	Wt loss > 5 % in 2 months or BMI 18.5–20.5 + impaired general condition or food intake 25–60 % of normal requirement in preceding week	Moderate **Score 2**	Major abdominal surgery; stroke; severe pneumonia; hematologic malignancy
Severe **Score 3**	Wt loss > 5 % in 1 month or BMI < 18.5 + impaired general condition or food intake below 50–70 % of normal requirement in preceding week	Severe **Score 3**	Head injury; bone marrow transplantation; intensive care patients (APACHE > 10)

Score: [Nutritional status score] + [Disease severity score] = **Total score**

Age If ≥ 70 years: add 1 to total score above = **Age-adjusted total score**

Score ≥ 3: the patient is nutritionally at risk and a nutritional care plan is initiated

Score < 3: weekly rescreening of the patient. If the patient, e.g., is scheduled for a major operation, a preventive nutritional care plan is considered to avoid the associated risk status

diets is somewhat controversial, the following considerations are generally accepted:

- Formulas containing arginine, omega-3 fatty acids, and nucleotides can reduce length of stay, rates of infection, and wound complications such as dehiscence [9].
- Consider starting immunonutrition 5 to 7 days prior to major elective surgery and continue for 5 to 7 days postoperatively.
- These formulas should not be used in patients with severe sepsis, pregnant patients, or transplant patients on immunosuppressants [9].

MANAGEMENT OF NUTRITION IMMEDIATELY PREOPERATIVELY

NPO Status Prior to Surgery

Patients are routinely made NPO after midnight on the day prior to surgery based on the long-standing belief that the stomach must be empty of food to prevent aspiration during induction of anesthesia, but there is little data to support such a prolonged period of fasting. Due to delays in operating room scheduling, patients often end up fasting twelve or more hours, which has been shown to increase insulin resistance [10]. The most recent guidelines from the American Society of Anesthesiologists (ASA) recommend "cessation of fried and fatty foods for eight hours prior to surgery, cessation of solid food six hours prior to surgery, and cessation of clear liquids two hours prior to surgery" [11]. Outpatients presenting for elective surgery can be instructed to follow these dietary guidelines prior to presenting for surgery. For inpatients, consultants should discuss with surgeons if they are comfortable permitting patients to have a more limited period of NPO.

POSTOPERATIVE MANAGEMENT

Traditionally, diet advancement following surgery occurs only after return of bowel function as evidenced by bowel sounds, flatus, or a bowel movement; however, there is no evidence that these indicators of bowel function truly correlate with bowel activity or tolerance of oral intake [12]. Prolonged NPO status may result in endothelial microvilli atrophy, increased risk of bowel dysfunction, and infection [13]. Enteral nutrition given within 24 h postoperatively has numerous documented benefits, including:

- Maintenance of intestinal mucosal barrier [12, 13]
- Decreased septic and infectious complications [12–14]
- Less weight loss after surgery [12]
- Improved wound healing [12, 14]
- Reduced insulin resistance [14]
- Improved muscle function [14]
- Reduced mortality [13, 14]
- Shorter length of hospital stay [13]

Evidence-based guidelines advise starting enteral feedings within 24 to 48 h postoperatively. Feeding into the small bowel may be best tolerated, as small bowel motility returns most quickly [12]. The consulting internist should recommend to the surgical team that patients be permitted to eat as soon as postoperative nausea resolves [13].

While enteral nutrition is preferred, parenteral nutrition (PN) may be required in patients with postoperative ileus. Aggressive parenteral nutrition support is only validated for malnourished patients. Since there is no outcome effect of short-term provision of PN, PN should be delayed until 5 to 7 days postoperatively (after a diet has been attempted and not tolerated or the diagnosis of an ileus has been confirmed) for patients who are well nourished at baseline. Additionally, PN should only be started if the anticipated duration of use is at least 7 days. Short-term provision of PN for less than 5 days does not improve patient outcomes and may increase risk for infectious complications [15].

REFERENCES

1. Haydock DA, Hill GL. Impaired wound healing in surgical patients with varying degrees of malnutrition. JPEN. 1986;10(6):550–4.
2. Garth AK, Newsome CM, Simmance N, et al. Nutritional status, nutrition practices and post-operative complications in patients with gastrointestinal cancer. J Hum Nutr Diet. 2010;23(4):393–401.
3. Donald RA, Perry EG, Wittert GA, et al. The plasma ACTH, AVP, CRH and catecholamine responses to conventional and laparoscopic cholecystectomy. Clin Endocrinol. 1993;38(6):609–16.
4. White JV, Guenter P, Jensen G, et al. Academy Malnutrition Work Group; A.S.P.E.N. Malnutrition Task Force; A.S.P.E.N. Board of Directors. Consensus statement: Academy of Nutrition and Dietetics and American Society for Parenteral and Enteral Nutrition: characteristics recommended for the identification and documentation of adult malnutrition (undernutrition). JPEN. 2012;36(3):275–83.
5. Kondrup J, Allison SP, Elia M, et al. ESPEN guidelines for nutrition screening 2002. Clin Nutr. 2003;22(4):415–21.
6. Weimann A, Braga M, Harsanyi L, et al. ESPEN Guidelines on enteral nutrition: surgery including organ transplantation. Clin Nutr. 2006;25(2):224–44.
7. Miller KR, Wischmeter PE, Taylor B, et al. An evidence-based approach to perioperative nutrition support in the elective surgery patient. JPEN. 2013;37(39S):39–50S.
8. McClave SA, Kozar R, Martindale RG, et al. Summary points and consensus recommendations from the North American surgical nutrition summit. JPEN. 2013;37(1S):99–105s.
9. Marik PE, Zaloga GP. Immunonutrition in high-risk surgical patients: a systematic review and analysis of the literature. JPEN. 2010;34(4):378–86.
10. Peres Pimenta G, Aguilar-Nascimento JE. Prolonged preoperative fasting in elective surgical patients: why should we reduce it? Nutr Clin Pract. http://ncp.sagepub.com/content/early/2013/12/10/0884533613514277. Accessed 18 Dec 2013.
11. American Society of Anesthesiologists Committee. Practice guidelines for preoperative fasting and the use of pharmacologic agents to reduce the risk of pulmonary aspiration: application to healthy patients undergoing elective procedures: an updated report by the American Society of Anesthesiologists Committee on Standards and Practice Parameters. Anesthesiology. 2011;114(3):495–511.
12. Warren J, Bhalla V, Cresci G. Postoperative diet advancement: surgical dogma vs. evidence-based medicine. Nutr Clin Pract. 2011;26(2):115–25.
13. Enomoto TM, Larson D, Martindale RG. Patients requiring perioperative nutritional support. Med Clin N Am. 2013;97(6):1181–200.
14. Lewis SJ, Andersen HK, Thomas S. Early enteral nutrition within 24 h of intestinal surgery versus later commencement of feeding: a systematic review and meta-analysis. J Gastrointest Surg. 2009;13(3):569–75.
15. Martindale RG, McClave SA, Vanek VW, et al. Guidelines for the provision and assessment of nutrition support therapy in the adult critically ill patient: Society of Critical Care Medicine and American Society for Parenteral and Enteral Nutrition. Crit Care Med. 2009;37(5):1–30.

Chapter 42
Patients with a Solid Organ Transplant

Christopher J. Wong

BACKGROUND

Patients with solid organ transplants are living longer, are increasing in number, and frequently undergo surgery that is unrelated to their transplant [1]. These patients may be many years out from transplantation, and while they still may require specialty care, they are often primarily managed by generalists. The perioperative medicine consultant should have a working knowledge of care of such patients.

Having a solid organ transplant does not automatically confer a higher risk of complications for non-transplant-related surgery. There is evidence that abdominal solid organ transplant recipients can safely undergo elective cardiac surgery [2]. Diverticular surgery may have similar risk to non-transplant patients if elective, but higher risk if urgent [3].

PREOPERATIVE EVALUATION

While prospective data are lacking, individual operative risk likely depends on the surgical complexity, degree of immunosuppression, and graft function. A basic transplant history should be obtained by the medicine consultant (see Table 42.1). Other key elements of the preoperative evaluation include:

- Immunosuppressive regimen: plan for perioperative management, especially if patients are expected to be NPO. Consult with pharmacist experienced with transplant patients.
- Corticosteroid use—maintenance dose, previous pulses of high-dose steroids for rejection, prior episodes of adrenal insufficiency with infection or procedures.

M.B. Jackson et al. (eds.), *The Perioperative Medicine Consult Handbook*, DOI 10.1007/978-3-319-09366-6_42,
© Springer International Publishing Switzerland 2015

TABLE 42.1 BASIC TRANSPLANT HISTORY

Information	Example
Transplanted organ, indication, and date of transplant	*Liver transplant for hepatitis C cirrhosis 3 years ago*
Status of transplanted organ:	
Current function	*Transaminases, liver synthetic function (bilirubin, INR, albumin), creatinine*
	Last liver biopsy
Presence of recurrent disease in the transplanted organ	*Hepatitis C viral load*
Prior episodes of rejection and increased immunosuppression	*One episode of rejection 2 years ago, treated with pulse steroids*
Function of other organs that may be affected by immunosuppressive regimen or transplanted organ dysfunction	*Mild chronic kidney disease from calcineurin inhibitor (tacrolimus)*

- For higher-risk surgeries or specific questions, involve the appropriate transplant/specialty service to evaluate the patient for a complete preoperative assessment, and plan for whether they will need to follow the patient postoperatively.

PERIOPERATIVE MANAGEMENT

GRAFT FUNCTION

- Follow for signs of graft dysfunction, which may include examination and laboratory monitoring (e.g., creatinine for renal transplant)
- Coordinate with transplant specialist when appropriate

MEDICATION MANAGEMENT

- Consider supplemental ("stress") dose steroids when indicated (see Chap. 14).
- Continue all usual immunosuppressant medications, including the morning of surgery.
- If patient receives prophylactic medications against opportunistic infections, continue them.
- If NPO postoperatively, convert antirejection medications to IV. Table 42.2 shows the general guidelines and recommendations for when to consult with a transplant pharmacist.

TABLE 42.2 COMMON ANTIREJECTION MEDICATIONS: PO TO IV CONVERSION

Cyclosporine	Give 1/3 of total daily PO dose as continuous infusion over 24 h (e.g., usual dose of 75 mg PO BID, total dose is 150 mg, 1/3 = 50 mg, can be given as 2.1 mg/h IV infusion). Monitor levels daily Note when converting back to oral cyclosporine, the common oral formulations Neoral® and Sandimmune® are *not* equivalent and should not be substituted for one another. It is best to maintain the patient's usual formulation and consult with a transplant pharmacist
Mycophenolate	Note different PO forms: mycophenolate mofetil (CellCept®, MMF) 500 mg = mycophenolate sodium (Myfortic®) 360 mg IV and PO dose of CellCept generally considered equivalent
Tacrolimus (FK506)	Often not given IV due to difficulty in titrating the dose—must consult with transplant pharmacist and organ specialty service as appropriate. They may recommend using cyclosporine instead

TABLE 42.3 COMMON DRUG INTERACTIONS WITH CYCLOSPORINE AND TACROLIMUS

Increase levels	Decrease levels
Erythromycin Azole antifungals Diltiazem Verapamil Metoclopramide Grapefruit juice	Rifampin Phenytoin Phenobarbital Carbamazepine

- Cyclosporine and tacrolimus have multiple drug interactions. A partial list is shown in Table 42.3. Review any new medication for possible interactions prior to starting it.
- Consider monitoring of immunosuppression in hospitalized patients to ensure therapeutic levels.
- Cyclosporine and tacrolimus can compromise renal function—avoid administration of nephrotoxic agents such as NSAIDs.
- Note that wound healing may be impaired in immunosuppressed patients. Sirolimus (Rapamune®) may cause a higher risk of wound complications; while this concern should be

alerted to the surgical team, any change in immunosuppression regimen should be made in discussion with the transplant/specialty service managing it.

INFECTION

- The immunosuppressed patient may not present with typical features of infection such as fever or leukocytosis.
- Patients who have well-functioning grafts greater than 6 months post-transplant tend to develop similar infections to patients without transplants. However, a poorly functioning graft or prior episodes of rejection are risk factors for opportunistic infections at any time.
- Infections may progress rapidly due to immunosuppression.
- Consultation with transplant team/infectious disease team is often appropriate when there is high suspicion of infection or an identified infection as adjustments may need to be made in the antibiotic or immunosuppressant regimen.

REFERENCES

1. Kostopanagiotu G, Smyrniotis V, Arkadopolous N. Anesthetic and perioperative management of adult transplant recipients in nontransplant surgery. Anesth Analg. 1999;89:613–22.
2. Ono M, Wolf RK, Angouras DC, et al. Short- and long-term results of open heart surgery in patients with abdominal solid organ transplant. Eur J Cardiothorac Surg. 2002;21:1061–72.
3. Reshef A, Stocchi L, Kiran RP, et al. Case-matched comparison of perioperative outcomes after surgical treatment of sigmoid diverticulitis in solid organ transplant recipients versus immunocompetent patients. Colorectal Dis. 2012;14:1546–52.

Chapter 43
Substance Abuse and Dependence

Ashok Reddy

BACKGROUND

Substance abuse and dependence pose several risks in the perioperative setting. For example, excessive alcohol use increases the risk of morbidity during surgery—including cardiopulmonary, infections, wound, bleeding, and neurologic complications [1]. Surgical patients who drink over four alcoholic drinks daily have a two- to threefold increased risk for postoperative complications when compared to patients who drink less than two drinks a day [3]. However, other than for alcohol, there are limited data for interventions to improve perioperative outcomes.

PREOPERATIVE EVALUATION

Patients should be assessed for substance abuse or dependence. There are various screening tools, including the AUDIT-C questionnaire, for alcohol abuse or dependence as shown in Table 43.1. Key points include:

- Higher scores on the AUDIT-C are associated with increases in postoperative complications [3, 4].
- In heavy alcohol users (five or more drinks a day), research demonstrated that 4 weeks of preoperative abstinence decreases the risk of postoperative complications [5].
- Acute withdrawal may contribute to postoperative morbidity and should be avoided if possible.

The use of illicit drugs is associated with pulmonary and cardiac complications that may affect management in the perioperative setting [6]. Identifying patients who abuse illegal drugs can be screened effec-

M.B. Jackson et al. (eds.), *The Perioperative Medicine Consult Handbook*, DOI 10.1007/978-3-319-09366-6_43,
© Springer International Publishing Switzerland 2015

TABLE 43.1 SCREENING ASSESSMENT: AUDIT-C QUESTIONNAIRE [2]

Question 1: "How often did you have a drink containing alcohol in the past 12 months?"

    Response (score): never (0), monthly or less (1), 2–4 times a month (2), 2–3 times a week (3), 4 or more a week (4)

Question 2: "How many drinks containing alcohol did you have on a typical day when you were drinking in the past 12 months?"

    Response (score): 0 drink (0), 1–2 drinks (0), 3–4 drinks (1), 5–6 drinks (2), 7–9 drinks (3), and 10 or more (4)

Question 3: "How often did you have 6 or more drinks on an occasion in the past 12 months?"

    Response (score): never (0), less than monthly (1), monthly (2), weekly (3), and daily (4)

AUDIT-C score is the sum of the points from each question (range 0–12 points)

tively using a single question: "How many times in the past year have you used an illegal drug or used a prescription medication for non-medical reasons?" In an urban primary care setting, this single screening question was 100 % sensitive and 73.5 % specific for the detection of a drug use disorder [7].

- An injection drug use history should prompt investigation for infectious or other complications.
- Active substance abuse or dependence identified during preoperative evaluation is an indication for referral to primary care and counseling or rehabilitation resources.

PERIOPERATIVE MANAGEMENT

Patients at risk for withdrawal during preoperative evaluation should have appropriate measures taken in the postoperative setting. Consideration of withdrawal syndromes is part of a full assessment of delirium in the postoperative setting (see Chap. 46). In some cases, patients have undergone emergency surgery and are unable to provide a history—additional information regarding substance use may need to be obtained from other sources. Patients identified with substance abuse or dependence should be referred to appropriate rehabilitation services. Withdrawal management strategies for specific substances are summarized below [8].

ALCOHOL
Withdrawal Signs and Symptoms
- Acute alcohol withdrawal generally starts 6 to 24 h after the patient takes the last drink of alcohol.
- Signs and symptoms include: restlessness, agitation, anxiety, nausea, vomiting, tremor, increased blood pressure, hyperthermia, delusions, delirium, and seizures.

Withdrawal Management
- Monitoring and treatment use Clinical Institute Withdrawal Assessment for Alcohol, revised (CIWA-Ar) paired with symptom-triggered use of benzodiazepines [9]

OPIOIDS
Withdrawal Signs and Symptoms
- Tachycardia, hypertension, hyperthermia, insomnia, enlarged pupils, diaphoresis, hyperreflexia, increased respiratory rate, abdominal cramps, nausea, vomiting, diarrhea, muscle pain, and anxiety

Withdrawal Management
- Consider monitoring and measuring opioid withdrawal using Subjective Opioid Withdrawal Scale (SOWS) and Objective Opioid Withdrawal Scale (OOWS) [10].
- The currently approved medications for management of opioid withdrawal include: methadone, clonidine, and buprenorphine. Consider consultation with a pharmacist for additional questions.

BENZODIAZEPINES AND OTHER SEDATIVE-HYPNOTICS
Withdrawal Signs and Symptoms
- Sleep disturbance, irritability, anxiety, panic attacks, tremors, nausea, vomiting, palpitations, headaches, potential delirium, and seizures

Withdrawal Management
- Current treatment recommendations are to begin a slow taper based on patient's assessed use of medications, consideration of switching to a benzodiazepine with a longer half-life (e.g., diazepam).
- In some cases phenobarbital substitution may be considered.

STIMULANTS (COCAINE AND AMPHETAMINES)
Withdrawal Signs and Symptoms
- Depression, insomnia, fatigue, anxiety, paranoia, and increased appetite

Withdrawal Management
- Withdrawal usually does not involve medical danger and management is based on patient symptoms.

MARIJUANA AND OTHER DRUGS CONTAINING THC-SUBSTANCES
Withdrawal Signs and Symptoms
- Irritability, aggression, depressed mood, restlessness, weight loss, headaches, sweating, fever, chills, and sweating

Withdrawal Management
- Withdrawal usually does not involve medical danger and management is based on patient symptoms.
- Evidence is limited on pharmacologic treatments for marijuana withdrawal.

REFERENCES

1. Tonnesen H, Kehlet H. Preoperative alcoholism and postoperative morbidity. Br J Surg. 1999;86:869–74.
2. Bush K, Kivlahan DR, McDonell MB, Fihn SD, Bradley KA. The AUDIT alcohol consumption questions (AUDIT-C): an effective brief screening test for problem drinking. Ambulatory Care Quality Improvement Project (ACQUIP). Alcohol Use Disorders Identification Test. Arch Intern Med. 1998;158:1789–95.
3. Bradley KA, Rubinsky AD, Sun H, Bryson CL, et al. Alcohol screening and risk of postoperative complications in male VA patients undergoing major non-cardiac surgery. J Gen Intern Med. 2011;26(2):162–9.
4. Rubinsky AD, et al. AUDIT-C alcohol screening results and postoperative inpatient health care use. J Am Coll Surg. 2012;214(3):296–305.
5. Tonnesen H, Rosenberg J, Nielsen H, et al. Effect of preoperative abstinence on poor postoperative in alcohol misusers: randomized controlled trial. BMJ. 1999;318(7194):1311–6.
6. Laine C, Williams SV, Wilson JF. In the clinic. Preoperative evaluation. Ann Intern Med. 2009;151(1):ITC1–15.
7. Smith PC, Schmidt SM, Allensworth-Davies D, Saitz R. A single-question screening test for drug use in primary care. Arch Intern Med. 2010;170(13):1155–60.
8. Center for Substance Abuse Treatment. Detoxification and Substance Abuse Treatment. Treatment Improvement Protocol (TIP) Series 45. DHHS Publication No. (SMA) 06-4131. Rockville, MD: Substance Abuse and Mental Health Services Administration; 2006.
9. Mayo-Smith MF. Pharmacological management of alcohol withdrawal: a meta-analysis and evidence-based practice guideline. JAMA. 1997;278(2):144–51.
10. Handelsman L, et al. Two new rating scales for opiate withdrawal. Am J Drug Alcohol Abuse. 1987;13(3):293–308.

Chapter 44
The Postoperative Evaluation

Nason P. Hamlin

BACKGROUND

Different hospitals have varying models regarding medical consultation. Some medicine consult services predominantly perform preoperative evaluations; others also work in the inpatient setting providing postoperative expertise. This section is for those medical consultants who provide care postoperatively.

POST-ANESTHESIA CARE UNIT ASSESSMENT

Assessing patients in the post anesthesia care unit (PACU) following surgery provides a great opportunity to avert problems and enhance continuity of care.

CHART REVIEW
- Pre-op evaluation: Review the patient's preoperative evaluation.
- Surgery: Did the patient receive the surgery that was planned, or were there unanticipated changes or complications?
- Check the estimated blood loss (EBL), amount and type of fluids received, and degree of hemodynamic stability intraoperatively—typically found in the anesthesia record or the operating note or directly from communication with the surgery or anesthesia teams.

M.B. Jackson et al. (eds.), *The Perioperative Medicine Consult Handbook*, DOI 10.1007/978-3-319-09366-6_44,
© Springer International Publishing Switzerland 2015

HISTORY AND PHYSICAL EXAM

Ask patients about chest pain, shortness of breath, nausea, and level of pain. Remember that patients are still coming out of anesthesia, so a negative response does not necessarily mean that there is no problem. For example, in an unstable patient at substantial risk for post-op MI, do not let a lack of chest pain steer you away from ordering an ECG and cardiac enzymes.

Patients often have limited mobility immediately on recovery from surgery and the physical examination may need to be adjusted.

Vital Signs

- Temperature: Postoperative patients are often hypothermic which increases their risk of complications. PACU nurses are usually attuned to this and will put a warming blanket or device on the patient.
- Blood pressure: Blood pressure can be quite labile as the effects of anesthesia are wearing off. Patients may have transient hypertension due to pain. Make sure that the pain is acceptably controlled before aggressive BP management. Shivering or tremors can also lead to a spuriously elevated BP reading on an automatic BP cuff. When in doubt, check it manually and in both arms.

MANAGEMENT
Common Items to Review

- Check the surgeon's orders to make sure that the medications are correct and that the recommendations in the preoperative evaluation are being followed.
- Diabetes management: Check insulin orders (see Chap. 13).
- Cardiovascular medications: Check for correct hold parameters for blood pressure meds and beta-blockers. Make sure that patients on beta-blockers pre-op for cardiovascular indications have them continued post-op (see Chap. 8).
- If you write orders (after discussion with the primary team), make sure to let the patient's nurse know. In hospitals that use paper chart orders, admission orders may already be sent to the nursing unit, and new orders may be missed. In hospitals that use computerized provider order entry (CPOE), orders may still be missed in transition and good communication remains essential during the transition from PACU to the nursing unit.
- If the patient's condition warrants a change in post-PACU care (e.g., requiring ICU or telemetry), make those recommendations and call the primary team.

DAILY POSTOPERATIVE EVALUATION

Common postoperative issues are discussed in greater detail throughout this handbook. General principles applicable to all postoperative patients include:

- Review interval history, examination, medication list, and labs/studies as you would for any medical patient.
- Review drains and catheters—these may not be as common in medical patients.
- What is the surgery team's plan? Discuss with the surgery team if in doubt.
- All patients: Is there appropriate VTE prophylaxis? (see Chap. 31).
- Lung expansion maneuvers: Are they indicated, and, if so, being done?
- Pay attention to side effects of pain medications and sedatives.
- Comment on each problem you are asked to evaluate, especially the medical concerns.
- Know the patient's current and anticipated bowel function status and whether they are able to receive PO medications.

NEW POSTOPERATIVE CONSULTS

For the new post-op consult, the above information still needs to be gathered. In addition, make sure of the following:

- Obtain the information for the requesting provider (name, service, contact number).
- Understand the clinical question clearly.
- Give the requesting provider a time frame in which you expect to see the patient and contact that provider.
- Review the surgery—were there complications? What were the duration, EBL, and method of anesthesia?
- Post-op course to date—have there been complications? Is the recovery going as expected? You should have a general sense of the length of stay, average blood loss, and recovery period for the procedure (see Chap. 48), and keep in mind that there may be site-specific and patient-specific differences. If in doubt, ask your surgical colleagues.

- You may need to seek other information—the patient may have post-op delirium or still be recovering from anesthesia. If you need a better history, you may need to seek out the patient's family, the surgeon, and nursing staff.
- The pre-op med list may not be accurate. You may need to double-check the patient's baseline meds.

Chapter 45
Postoperative Fever

Kara J. Mitchell

BACKGROUND

Postoperative fever is a common finding [1]. While most early fever is due to cytokine release and resolves spontaneously [2], the possibility of infection should be at least considered in most cases of postoperative fever. Remember, patients may have infection in the absence of fever, especially with advanced age, corticosteroid use, and other risk factors; infection may occasionally present with hypothermia [1].

PERIOPERATIVE MANAGEMENT

STRATEGIES TO PREVENT POSTOPERATIVE INFECTION

- Stop unnecessary medications, especially antibiotics. After most uncomplicated surgeries, prophylactic antibiotics should be discontinued within 24 h of surgery.
- Discontinue catheters (Foley, nasogastric tube, central lines, etc.) as soon as possible. For example, guidelines recommend discontinuing a urethral catheter within 24 h of surgery unless there are indications for it to remain in place: acute urinary retention, critically ill patients requiring accurate measurements, open sacral or perineal wounds in incontinent patients, prolonged immobilization, and end-of-life care [3].

M.B. Jackson et al. (eds.), *The Perioperative Medicine Consult Handbook*, DOI 10.1007/978-3-319-09366-6_45,
© Springer International Publishing Switzerland 2015

- The femoral site should be avoided for central venous catheters. The subclavian site is recommended over the internal jugular to minimize infection risk, but site-specific complication risk should be considered, in addition to infection control [4].
- Implement a plan to reduce ventilator-associated pneumonia, including sedation vacations, weaning plan, and semi-upright head positioning.
- Use enteral nutrition, when possible, instead of total parenteral nutrition.

EVALUATION OF PATIENTS WITH POSTOPERATIVE FEVER

Immediate causes of fever include cytokine release, medications, and transfusion reactions. Atelectasis does not cause fever; it can cause hypoxia and should still be treated [2, 5]. Watch for life-threatening causes of early fever such as malignant hyperthermia, neuroleptic malignant syndrome, serotonin syndrome, necrotizing fasciitis, toxic shock syndrome, transfusion reaction, etc. After 48 h, important considerations include surgical site infections, pneumonia, urinary tract infections, catheter infections, and many noninfectious causes [6]. Timing of onset of fever is a major key to determining its cause (see Table 45.1).

Cultures have little utility in the first 48 h after surgery, unless there is suspicion for antecedent infection. Fever occurring after postoperative day 3, multiple days of fever, and maximum temperature of greater than or equal to 39C are predictors of a positive fever evaluation [7]. A brief bedside evaluation has the highest yield for determining the etiology of a fever [8]. After 72 h, consider ordering the following tests, using the bedside evaluation and the clinical context as a guide [1, 6]:

- CBC with differential ± other blood tests, as indicated by the situation
- Blood culture when fever is present (draw two sets peripherally or one from the central line and one from the peripheral line)
- Urinalysis, Gram stain, and urine culture. If urinary catheter is present, ideally remove catheter and obtain a clean catch specimen; if unable to remove the catheter, then obtain sample from the catheter port (not the urine bag)
- Chest X-ray ± sputum Gram stain and culture, if pneumonia suspected
- Tap fluid collections, as appropriate (pleural, peritoneal, joint, CSF, etc.)
- Appropriate imaging (i.e., CT or ultrasound for abdominal pain, CT pulmonary angiogram if pulmonary embolism is suspected, ECG if concern for myocardial infection, etc.)
- Stool for C. difficile if suspicious diarrhea and recent antibiotics

TABLE 45.1 CAUSES OF POSTOPERATIVE FEVER BY TIME AFTER SURGERY

Immediate (within hours)	Acute (within the first week)	Subacute (1–4 weeks out)
Trauma/cytokine release	Surgical site infection (after 48 h)	Surgical site infection
Medications, including malignant hyperthermia	Pneumonia	Thrombophlebitis/ DVT/PE
Transfusion reaction	UTI	*C. difficile*
Necrotizing fasciitis	IV catheter infection	Drug reaction[a]
Infection, thrombosis, or other noninfectious causes present prior to surgery	Noninfectious: MI, DVT/PE, CVA/SAH, thrombophlebitis, hematoma, pancreatitis, alcohol withdrawal, gout, bowel ischemia, TTP, hyperthyroidism, adrenal insufficiency, transfusion or medication reaction, inflammatory reaction to implanted hardware, etc.	Nosocomial or other infections: pneumonia, UTI, IV catheter-related infection, intra-abdominal abscess, sinusitis, otitis media, osteomyelitis, endocarditis, cholecystitis (can be acalculous), etc.[b] [Neoplasia and collagen-vascular diseases are less common causes of postoperative fever]

[a]Commonly implicated medications: beta-lactams, sulfa, phenytoin, heparin, etc. [6]

[b]Watch for surgery-specific causes: i.e., meningitis after neurosurgery, toxic shock after nasal or vaginal packing, parotitis after oral surgery, rejection after transplant surgery, fat emboli after orthopedic surgery, infected hardware or graft material, etc.

TREATMENT OF POSTOPERATIVE FEVER

The mainstay of management of postoperative fever is the identification and treatment of the underlying cause. Several principles should be kept in mind:

- Avoid empiric antibiotics unless there is a specific indication: neutropenic fever, hemodynamic instability, or suspicion of a high-risk diagnosis such as meningitis.
- If empiric antibiotics are given, stop or narrow these after 48 h if the patient is stable and cultures remain sterile.

- Infected wounds and fluid collections require debridement and/or drainage.
- Acetaminophen may be given for comfort (risk of hepatotoxicity with liver disease or starvation); use aspirin and NSAIDs only with caution (risk of renal failure, GI ulceration, or wound bleeding) [9].

REFERENCES

1. O'Grady NP, Barie PS, Bartlett JG, et al. Guidelines for evaluation of new fever in critically ill adult patients: 2008 update from the American College of Critical Care Medicine and the Infectious Diseases Society of America. Crit Care Med. 2008;36:1330–49.
2. Netea MG, Kullberg BJ, Van der Meer JW. Circulating cytokines as mediators of fever. Clin Infect Dis. 2000;31:S178–84.
3. Gould CV, Umscheid CA, Agarwal RK, et al. Guideline for prevention of catheter-associated urinary tract infections 2009. Healthcare Infection Control Practices Advisory Committee, CDC. http://www.cdc.gov/hicpac/pdf/CAUTI/CAUTIguideline2009final.pdf
4. Grady NP, Alexander M, Burns LA, et al. Guidelines for the prevention of intravascular catheter-related infections. CDC; 2011. http://www.cdc.gov/hicpac/pdf/guidelines/bsiguidelines-2011.pdf
5. Mavros MN, Velmahos GC, Falagas ME. Atelectasis as a cause of postoperative fever: where is the clinical evidence? Chest. 2011;140:418–24.
6. Weed HG, Baddour LM. Postoperative fever. UpToDate, Basow DS (Ed), UpToDate, Waltham, MA. Accessed 25 Jan 2014.
7. Ward ET, et al. Cost and effectiveness of postoperative fever diagnostic evaluation in total joint arthroplasty patients. J Arthroplasty. 2010;25:43–8.
8. Lesperancne R, et al. Early postoperative fever and the "Routine" fever work-up: results of a prospective study. J Surg Res. 2011;171:245–50.
9. Plaisance KI, Mackowiak PA. Antipyretic therapy: physiologic rationale, diagnostic implications, and clinical consequences. Arch Intern Med. 2000;160:449–56.

Chapter 46
Postoperative Delirium

Andrew A. White and Tyler Lee

BACKGROUND

Delirium is a common and serious altered mental state that may develop due to a wide variety of medical conditions or drug side effects. It is characterized by the following:

1. Acute onset and fluctuating course
2. Inattention
3. Disorganized thinking or a change in cognition
4. Altered level of consciousness

Using the confusion assessment method (CAM), delirium is most reliably diagnosed by the presence of the first two findings and at least one of the last two [1]. According to the DSM-V definition, it may also be accompanied by sleep-wake cycle disturbance and shifting emotional disturbances [2]. Hypoactive delirium may be missed due to subtle manifestations. The pathogenesis of delirium is poorly understood and most likely multifactorial. Delirium may occur in up to 70 % of post-surgery patients [3], but the incidence varies widely with both patient- and surgery-specific risk factors. Meta-analyses have produced the estimates of incidence shown in Table 46.1. Perioperative delirium is associated with greater cost, longer length of stay, greater morbidity, increased likelihood of subsequent institutionalization, prolonged functional decline, and mortality [6].

PREOPERATIVE EVALUATION

Certain patient populations are inherently vulnerable to developing delirium. In addition, the duration and physiologic stress of the surgery influence the likelihood of precipitating delirium. Inherent risk

M.B. Jackson et al. (eds.), *The Perioperative Medicine Consult Handbook*, DOI 10.1007/978-3-319-09366-6_46, © Springer International Publishing Switzerland 2015

TABLE 46.1 ESTIMATES OF INCIDENCE OF DELIRIUM IN INPATIENTS

Type of surgery/reason for admission	Incidence of delirium
ICU care (surgical and medical patients >65 years old) [3]	70–87 %
Elective vascular surgery [1, 2]	34.5 % (29–39 %)
Cardiac surgery [4]	32 % (0–73 %)
Hip fracture [5]	21.7 % (4–53 %)
Elective hip or knee replacement [3]	12.1 % (9–28 %)
Major elective surgery [1, 2]	10 % (9–17 %)

TABLE 46.2 PATIENT RISK FACTORS FOR DELIRIUM

Age > 65	Cognitive dysfunction, especially dementia
Prior stroke	Prior history of delirium
Depression	Reduced preoperative functional status
Vision and hearing impairment	Preoperative psychotropic drug use
HIV	Drug and alcohol abuse
Renal or liver disease	Male gender
Malnutrition	

factors are shown in Table 46.2 [1, 2]. Cardiopulmonary bypass may be a surgery-specific risk factor for delirium associated with more protracted cognitive dysfunction, but studies in this area are heterogeneous. Current evidence suggests it is most important to focus on reducing patient-specific risk factors, rather than the form of surgery or anesthesia [7].

PERIOPERATIVE MANAGEMENT

PREVENTION

Prevention trials utilizing behavioral and environmental approaches have demonstrated a reduction in delirium incidence (absolute risk reduction 5–18 %) [8, 9]. Geriatrics consultation has also been shown to be helpful [9]. Pharmacologic prevention trials in high-risk patients have not consistently shown a reduction in delirium incidence, but may affect duration and severity. In the absence of better data,

TABLE 46.3 PREVENTION OF DELIRIUM IN POSTOPERATIVE PATIENTS

Providing visual and hearing aids when appropriate

Early mobilization

Avoid volume depletion and electrolyte abnormalities

Discontinue or substitute high-risk medications

Frequent reorientation

Maintain day/night cycle by limiting naps, opening blinds, avoiding nighttime interruptions

Adequate pain control without oversedation

Consider geriatric consultation

prophylactic antipsychotics are not warranted for most patients [10]. Anticholinesterase inhibitors have not been shown to effectively prevent delirium. During postoperative ICU care, the use of dexmedetomidine instead of benzodiazepines for sedation has been associated with lower rates of delirium, but is more costly and associated with bradycardia [11]. Effective prevention strategies are shown in Table 46.3.

DIAGNOSIS

First, confirm the diagnosis of delirium by excluding other neurologic and psychiatric conditions. Then, focus on identifying precipitants with history, medication review, physical exam (particularly neurologic and cognitive exam), and basic lab tests (CBC, Chem 7, UA). When appropriate, ECG, CXR, drug levels, or a toxin screen may confirm a suspected etiology. Remember that the etiology may be multifactorial. Head CT scan is often not helpful unless there is a risk factor for intracranial bleeding (e.g., history of fall or anticoagulant use) or evidence of new focal neurologic impairment.

PRECIPITATING ETIOLOGIES

Many medications and medical conditions can contribute to the development of delirium. Among frail elderly patients, delirium is commonly a multifactorial syndrome without a clear single etiology. Although the following list is not comprehensive, consider the following common precipitants:

- *Medications*: anesthetic agents, sedative-hypnotics, barbiturates, alcohol, antidepressants, anticholinergics, opioid analgesics, antipsychotics, anticonvulsants, antihistamines, corticosteroids, fluoroquinolones, and antiparkinsonian agents. Also be wary of polypharmacy.

TABLE 46.4 TREATMENT OF DELIRIUM

Supportive care Delirium can lead to injury or irreversible functional decline Prevention of such sequelae includes the following steps	Optimize nutrition and avoid dehydration
	Mobilize frequently to prevent pressure ulcers and functional decline
	Prevent aspiration with head of bed precautions when appropriate
	Optimize bowel regimen
	Fall and wander precautions when appropriate
	Treat pain, hypoxia, and hypercarbia
Behavioral control The first principle of behavioral management is to utilize environmental or social measures rather than pharmacologic or physical restraints whenever possible	Frequent orientation, including posting of calendar and clock
	Involve family and consistent providers to provide familiar context
	Maintain night/day cycle
	Constant observer or wander guard
	Consider securing or protecting vulnerable lines, drains, and wounds from harmful manipulation
Pharmacologic treatment If behavioral interventions fail or agitated, delirium is life-threatening (such as in the ICU), consider the following	Low-dose haloperidol (0.5–1 mg PO/IM/IV q bedtime to bid PRN)
	Risperidone (0.5 mg PO q 12 h PRN) is an acceptable alternative
	Recall that these are contraindicated in patients with neuroleptic malignant syndrome, prolonged QTc, or parkinsonism
	Reassess behavior frequently and stop the antipsychotic medication a few days after delirium has resolved
	Benzodiazepines often worsen confusion and sedation and should typically be avoided for behavior management

- *Acute medical conditions*: fluid, electrolyte and metabolic abnormalities (sodium, glucose, calcium, urea), vitamin deficiency (thiamine), uncontrolled pain, hypoxemia, hypercarbia, fever, hypotension, anemia, infections (UTI, pneumonia, line infections), myocardial infarction, alcohol and drug withdrawal, constipation, and urinary retention.

- *Iatrogenic*: sleep cycle disruption, catheters and other "tethers" (IV lines, ECG leads, and restraints), and lack of access to hearing aids, glasses, interpreter services, food, and water.

TREATMENT

Delirium is typically reversible if the precipitating factors are addressed. Identifying and treating underlying causes of delirium are essential for recovery. Simultaneously, consider ways to provide supportive care and, if necessary, manage behavioral symptoms. Due to methodological limitations, existing studies do not support the use of antipsychotics in the treatment of delirium [12]. However, antipsychotics may play a limited role in the management of behavioral or emotional symptoms. Second-generation antipsychotics are not superior to haloperidol, except when there is concern for extrapyramidal symptoms or QTc prolongation [13]. Treatment recommendations are shown in Table 46.4.

REFERENCES

1. Inouye SK, van Dyck CH, Alessi CA, et al. Clarifying confusion: the confusion assessment method. Ann Intern Med. 1990;113:941–8.
2. American Psychiatric Association. Diagnostic and statistical manual of mental disorders. 5th ed. Arlington, VA: American Psychiatric Association; 2013.
3. Dyer CB, Ashton CM, Teasdale TA. Postoperative delirium. A review of 80 primary data-collection studies. Arch Intern Med. 1995;155(5):461–5.
4. Sockalingam S, Parekh N, Bogoch I, et al. Delirium in the postoperative cardiac patient: a review. J Card Surg. 2005;20(6):560–7.
5. Bruce AJ, Ritchie CW, Blizard R, et al. The incidence of delirium associated with orthopedic surgery: a meta-analytic review. Int Psychogeriatr. 2007;19(2):197–214.
6. Dasgupta M, Dumbrell A. Preoperative risk assessment for delirium after noncardiac surgery: a systemic review. J Am Geriatr Soc. 2006;54:1578–89.
7. Selnes OA, Gottesman RF, Grega MA, et al. Cognitive and neurologic outcomes after coronary-artery bypass surgery. N Engl J Med. 2012;366:250–7.
8. Inouye SK, Bogardus ST, Charpentier PA, et al. A multicomponent intervention to prevent delirium in hospitalized older patients. N Engl J Med. 1999;340:669–76.
9. Marcantonio ER, Flacker JM, Wright JR, et al. Reducing delirium after hip fracture: a randomized trial. J Am Geriatr Soc. 2001;49(5):516–22.
10. Kalisvaart KJ, deJonghe JF, Bogaards MJ, et al. Haloperidol prophylaxis for elderly hip-fracture patients at risk for delirium: a randomized, placebo-controlled study. J Am Geriatr Soc. 2005;53(10):1658–66.
11. Riker RR, et al. Dexmedetomidine vs midazolam for sedation of critically ill patients. A randomized trial. JAMA. 2009;301(5):489–99.
12. Flaherty JH, Gonzales JP, Dong B. Antipsychotics in the treatment of delirium in older hospitalized adults: a systematic review. J Am Geriatr Soc. 2011;59:S269–76.
13. Campbell N, Boustani M, Ayub A, et al. Pharmacological management of delirium in hospitalized older adults—a systematic review. J Gen Intern Med. 2009;24(7):848–53.

Chapter 47
Postoperative Ileus

Sandra M. Demars

BACKGROUND

It is normal for patients postoperatively to have "physiologic" gastrointestinal (GI) tract dysmotility. Some degree of dysmotility is expected in all patients following intra-abdominal surgery. Without treatment, it is expected to last 3–6 days following major abdominal surgery [1, 2]. GI tract dysmotility may also occur following thoracic, orthopedic, urologic, and gynecologic operations if somatovisceral reflexes are activated intraoperatively [2].

Ileus, on the other hand, is the state of prolonged dysmotility beyond the expected time frame. As one of the most common postsurgical complications, ileus occurs in 3–30 % of patients following various types of abdominal operations [3]. Clinically, this manifests as the absence of flatus or bowel movement; abdominal distension associated with pain, nausea, and emesis; and the inability to tolerate oral intake. This not only increases patient discomfort, dissatisfaction, and immobility but also increases hospital stay duration by 4–6 days thereby increasing direct health-care costs by approximately $9,000 per hospital stay [3, 4]. The economic consequences of postoperative ileus (POI) following abdominal surgery on the US health-care system are estimated to reach close to $1.5 billion annually [3].

It is unknown why physiological postoperative GI tract dysmotility progresses to POI in some patients. It is likely a multifactorial process, and several mechanisms have been suggested, including autonomic nervous system dysfunction, inhibitory autonomic neural reflexes, inflammatory cytokines, gastrointestinal neurohumoral peptides, systemic opioids, and surgical technique [1, 2].

M.B. Jackson et al. (eds.), *The Perioperative Medicine Consult Handbook*, DOI 10.1007/978-3-319-09366-6_47,
© Springer International Publishing Switzerland 2015

PREOPERATIVE EVALUATION

It is difficult to predict which patients will develop POI, but the medicine consultant can anticipate that selected patients are at increased risk and should consider initiating preventative strategies. The following risk factors for POI have been identified:

- Longer operative times [5, 6]
- Excessive intraoperative small bowel manipulation/bowel resection surgery [6, 7]
- Perioperative decrease in hemoglobin or perioperative transfusion [5]
- Greater duration of nasogastric (NG) tube use [6, 7]
- Greater use of systemic opiates [5–7]
- Electrolyte abnormalities [7]
- Inadequate or excessive fluid resuscitation [7]

PERIOPERATIVE MANAGEMENT

EFFECTIVE STRATEGIES TO PREVENT POI

- *Epidural local anesthetic*: Mid-thoracic infusion for 2–3 days postoperatively reduces spinal inhibitory neural reflexes to the gut, thereby blunting the surgical stress response and decreasing the need for systemic opiates, and has been shown to accelerate the return of bowel function by 1–2 days [8]. This intervention has mostly been studied with intra-abdominal surgeries including vascular, gynecologic, and urologic procedures.
- *Alvimopan* (peripherally acting mu-opioid receptor antagonist): Multiple trials have shown decreased time to first stool and tolerance of diet, as well as shortened hospital stay durations [9]. However, due to concern for cardiovascular and neoplastic adverse effects, its use is currently limited to short-term use (15 doses), particular hospitals, and only to patients following bowel resection with primary anastomosis.
- *Postoperative gum chewing*: Meta-analyses reveal shortened time to first flatus and stool and decreased length of stay, with no increase in complications [10].
- *Avoidance/reduction of systemic opioids*: Opiate use increases the risk of POI [5]; acetaminophen, NSAIDs, tramadol, and

other non-opioid pain medications can minimize the need for opioids. NSAIDs must be used with caution due to potential gastrointestinal and renal toxicity. Preemptive use of medications to prevent central sensitization, such as gabapentin and dexamethasone, appears to be effective in minimizing postoperative pain if initiated before surgery [11, 12].

- *Multimodal surgical fast-track programs*: Programs used in elective colon surgery show that thoracic epidural analgesia combined with laxatives, early feeding, and early mobilization can achieve normal bowel function within 48 h postoperatively [13].

POTENTIALLY EFFECTIVE STRATEGIES TO PREVENT POI

- *Minimally invasive and minimally traumatic surgical techniques*: Laparoscopic surgery is associated with a shorter time to recovery of bowel function although it is not clear if this is because of the technique itself or because patients need less opiate pain control postoperatively [14].
- *Laxative use*: Data are limited but suggest benefit with no obvious harm. One trial following hysterectomy found the scheduled use of magnesium oxide laxative significantly minimized time to first bowel movement [15].
- *Restrictive fluid management*: One study showed that restrictive fluid management shortened duration of POI [7].
- *Postoperative coffee consumption*: One small study showed earlier time to first flatus and first bowel movement following open colectomy with postoperative coffee consumption [16].

UNPROVEN STRATEGIES TO PREVENT POI

- *Early postoperative feeding*: Some patients may suffer nausea or vomiting, but overall, early feeding does not appear harmful and may reduce the length of the hospital stay [17].
- *Early mobilization*: Only one study has evaluated early ambulation and it did not find earlier time to bowel recovery [18].
- *Promotility agents*: Metoclopramide, erythromycin, and neostigmine have not shown any benefit [1]. Cisapride, however, did show benefit but has been pulled from the US market because of reports of cardiac arrhythmias [1].
- *Various approaches currently under investigation* include methylnaltrexone, vagal stimulation, intravenous ghrelin, carbon monoxide, and pantothenic acid [1, 19–22].

EVALUATION OF PATIENTS WITH SUSPECTED POI
History and Physical Examination

Patient with POI will often complain of diffuse abdominal pain/distension, nausea, and emesis, inability to pass flatus or stool, or inability to tolerate a normal diet. Beware of signs suggesting bowel ischemia or perforation (fever, tachycardia, or peritoneal signs) that require emergent surgical evaluation. As the consultant evaluates the patient, alternative diagnoses should be considered including gastroparesis in patients with long-standing diabetes, and small bowel obstruction (SBO) in patients with previous abdominal surgeries, areas of potential hernia formation, abdominal masses, large tumor burden, stomas, or Crohn's disease. SBO should also be considered in the case of patients with intense colicky pain or feculent emesis. Other possible etiologies to consider in the differential diagnosis include constipation/stool impaction, acute colonic pseudo-obstruction, toxic megacolon, volvulus, anastomotic leak, and large bowel obstruction. Also be mindful of etiologies of secondary ileus, such as medications or other medical conditions, as discussed below.

Review the medication list for possible contributors to ileus:

- Opiates
- Anticholinergics
- Antihistamines
- Steroids
- Tricyclic antidepressants
- Calcium channel blockers
- H2 blockers

Common exam findings for POI include:

- Decreased, or absent, bowel sounds
- Abdominal distension
- Mild diffuse tenderness
- Tympany

Laboratory and Imaging Workup

Labs should be obtained to identify reversible factors leading to a secondary ileus, such as those listed below. Correction of the primary underlying problem should be treatment enough to resolve the secondary ileus.

- Leukocytosis: Consider sepsis, abdominopelvic abscess, cholecystitis, appendicitis, or bowel ischemia secondary to SBO.
- Hemoglobin/hematocrit: Consider intra-abdominal or retroperitoneal bleeding if decreased; consider dehydration if elevated.
- Chemistry panel: Evaluate for electrolyte imbalances that can cause ileus including hypokalemia, hypomagnesemia, hypona-

tremia, hypocalcemia, and uremia; consider sepsis or bowel ischemia secondary to SBO in the case of metabolic acidosis.
- Elevated liver function panel: Consider gallstones or pancreatitis.
- Elevated amylase/lipase: Consider pancreatitis.

Imaging should begin with supine and upright plain abdominal radiographs ("obstruction series") to distinguish between ileus and other pathologies. Common patterns include:
- Dilated loops of bowel (>3 cm): Seen in ileus or SBO.
- Paucity of gas in the colon: Seen in ileus or SBO.
- Air-fluid levels suggests SBO but may also be seen in ileus.
- Pneumoperitoneum: Concerning for bowel perforation or recent insufflation during laparoscopy. On supine films, look for Rigler's sign (double wall sign) which is a sign of lucency (gas) on both sides of the bowel wall. On upright films, look for free air under the diaphragm.
- Mucosal thickening (thumbprint sign) suggests bowel inflammation; concerning for bowel ischemia.
- Large bowel dilatation (>6 cm or >9 cm at the cecum) suggests large bowel obstruction or acute colonic pseudo-obstruction.
- Dilation of transverse colon/splenic flexure >6 cm, with alteration of normal wall contour (effacement or thumbprinting), intraluminal gas, and possibly pneumoperitoneum: Concerning for toxic megacolon.
- Dilated twisted loop of colon (coffee bean sign): Seen in volvulus.

Plain films, however, are often indeterminate. If you have clinical suspicion for a more serious problem, consider obtaining a CT abdomen/pelvis with oral contrast. Abdominal CT can also often identify secondary causes of ileus, such as abscess. If diagnosis after CT is still uncertain, consider upper gastrointestinal contrast studies with water-soluble contrast.

TREATMENT OF POI
- NPO except sips of clears.
- Intravenous fluid (IVF) as needed.
- Replete electrolytes as needed.
- Treat any constipation with appropriate agents.
- Replace gastrointestinal fluid losses with attention to electrolytes.
- Minimize opiates as able, and consider scheduled acetaminophen, tramadol, and judicious NSAID use (avoiding gastrointestinal and renal toxicity).
- Perform serial clinical evaluations and reimage for worsening or persistence.

- Do not routinely place an nasogastric (NG) tube, but if the patient has significant vomiting, distension, or pain, consider inserting one and putting it on low-intermittent wall suction (after checking with the surgical team to ensure that it is safe to do so).

- Once bowel function resumes, remove the NG tube (if present) and advance the diet as tolerated, beginning with clear liquids.

REFERENCES

1. Stewart D, Waxman K. Management of postoperative ileus. Dis Mon. 2010;56(4):204–14.
2. Miedema BW, Johnson JO. Methods for decreasing postoperative gut dysmotility. Lancet Oncol. 2003;4:365–72.
3. Goldstein JL, Matuszewski KA, Kelaney CP, et al. Inpatient economic burden of postoperative ileus associated with abdominal surgery in the United States. P&T. 2007;32(2):82-90. Available at http://www.ptcommunity.com/ptjournal/fulltext//32/2/PTJ3202082.pdf. Accessed 15 Jan 2014
4. Iver S, Saunders WB, Stemkowski S. Economic burden of postoperative ileus associated with colectomy in the United States. J Manag Care Pharm. 2009;15(6):485–94.
5. Artinyan A, Nunoo-Mensah JW, Balasubramaniam S, Gauderman J, Essani R, Gonzalez-Ruiz C, Kaiser AM, Beart Jr RW. Prolonged postoperative ileus-definition, risk factors, and predictors after surgery. World J Surg. 2008;32(7):1495–500.
6. Ay AA, Kutun S, Ulucanlar H, Tarcan O, Demir A, Cetin A. Risk factors for postoperative ileus. J Korean Surg Soc. 2011;81:242–9.
7. Vather R, Bissett I. Management of prolonged postoperative ileus: evidence-based recommendations. ANZ J Surg. 2013;83:319–24.
8. Jørgensen H, Wetterslev J, Møiniche S, Dahl JB. Epidural local anaesthetics versus opioid-based analgesic regimens on postoperative gastrointestinal paralysis, PONV and pain after abdominal surgery. Cochrane Database Syst Rev. 2000;(4):CD001893
9. Vaughan-Shaw PG, Fecher IC, Harris S, Knight JS. A meta-analysis of the effectiveness of the opioid receptor antagonist alvimopan in reducing hospital length of stay and time to GI recovery in patients enrolled in a standardized accelerated recovery program after abdominal surgery. Dis Colon Rectum. 2012;55:611–20.
10. Noble EJ, Harris R, Hosie KB, Thomas S, Lewis SJ. Gum chewing reduces postoperative ileus? A systematic review and meta-analysis. Int J Surg. 2009;7(2):100–5.
11. Pandey CK, Priye S, Singh S, Singh U, Singh RB, Singh PK. Preemptive use of gabapentin significantly decreases postoperative pain and rescue analgesic requirements in laparoscopic cholecystectomy. Can J Anaesth. 2004;51(4):358.
12. Bisgaard T, Klarshov B, Kehlet H, Rosenberg J. Preoperative dexamethasone improves surgical outcomes after laparoscopic cholecystectomy: a randomized double-blind placebo-controlled trial. Ann Surg. 2003;238(5):651.
13. Wind J, Polle SW, Fung Kon Jin PH, Dejong CH, von Meyenfeldt MF, Ubbink DT, Gouma DJ, Bemelman WA. Systematic review of enhanced recovery programs in colonic surgery. Br J Surg. 2006;93:800–9.
14. Abraham NS, Young JM, Solomon MJ. Meta-analysis of short-term outcomes after laparoscopic resection for colorectal cancer. Br J Surg. 2004;91(9):1111–24.
15. Hansen CT, Sørensen M, Møller C, Ottesen B, Kehlet H. Effect of laxatives on gastrointestinal functional recovery in fast-track hysterectomy: a double-blind, placebo-controlled randomized study. Am J Obstet Gynecol. 2007;196(4):311.e1–7.
16. Muller SA, Rahbari NN, Schmied BM, Buchler MW. Can postoperative coffee perk up recovery time after colon surgery? Expert Rev Gastroenterol Hepatol. 2013;7(2):91–3.
17. Mangesi L, Hofmeyr GJ. Early compared with delayed oral fluids and food after caesarean section. Cochrane Database Syst Rev. 2002;(3):CD003516.
18. Waldhausen JH, Schirmer BD. The effect of ambulation on recovery from postoperative ileus. Ann Surg. 1990;212(6):671.
19. Lubbers T, Buurman W, Luyer M. Controlling postoperative ileus by vagal activation. World J Gastroenterol. 2010;16(14):1683–7.

20. Falken Y, Webb DL, Abraham-Nordling M, Kressner U, Hellstrom PM, Naslund E. Intravenous ghrelin accelerates postoperative gastric emptying and time to first bowel movement in humans. Neurogastroenterol Motil. 2013;25(6):474–80.
21. Gibbons SJ, Verhulst PJ, Bharucha A, Farrugia G. Review article: carbon monoxide in gastrointestinal physiology and its potential in therapeutics. Aliment Phamacol Ther. 2013;38(7):689–702.
22. Giraldi G, De Luca d'Alessandro E, Mannocci A, Vecchione V, Martinoli L. A pilot study of the effects of pantothenic acid in the treatment of postoperative ileus: results from an orthopedic surgical department. Clin Ter. 2012;163(3):e121–6.

Chapter 48
Surgical Procedures Overview

Molly Blackley Jackson, Elizabeth Kaplan, Kara J. Mitchell, and Christina Ryan

BACKGROUND

The following sections describe typical, uncomplicated postoperative courses for a variety of surgeries. The details are presented from a medical, rather than a surgical, point of view. Our goal is to give the internist a general sense of the typical postoperative course and to highlight surgical issues that may impact other medical diagnoses and treatments. Every postoperative course is unique, however, and there is no substitute for communicating with an individual patient's surgical team.

ORTHOPEDIC SURGERY

TOTAL KNEE ARTHROPLASTY

2 h general anesthesia (GA) or regional/EBL: Less than 100 mL during procedure but can be quite high (500–1,500 mL) over first post-op day into drains (or into the knee, if no drains).

POD 0: IVF, diet advanced. PCA and/or regional anesthesia (femoral block or catheter) and Foley. Usually able to restart PO meds.

POD 1: Diet advanced if not yet done. Stop IV fluids if doing well with oral intake. Knee range of motion emphasized. Out of bed and walking with PT. Foley out. Transition from PCA to PO pain meds. VTE prophylaxis.

POD 2–3: D/C to home. Extended VTE prophylaxis on discharge.

M.B. Jackson et al. (eds.), *The Perioperative Medicine Consult Handbook*, DOI 10.1007/978-3-319-09366-6_48,
© Springer International Publishing Switzerland 2015

Tips

- Minimally invasive total knee arthroplasty (TKA) (MIS or quad sparing) may discharge earlier.
- Continuous passive motion (CPM) machine is sometimes used.
- Most primary (and some revision) TKAs are weight bearing as tolerated (WBAT).
- Common issues to TKAs and total hip arthroplasties (THAs): See below.

TOTAL HIP ARTHROPLASTY

2 h/GA or regional/EBL 300 mL (varies).

POD 0: IVF, diet advanced. PCA and Foley. Usually able to restart PO meds.

POD 1: Diet advanced if not yet done. Stop IV fluids if doing well with oral intake. Remove drain (if used) and Foley catheter if possible. Consider transition to PO pain meds. VTE prophylaxis.

POD 2–3: Stop PCA, change to PO pain meds if not already done. Extended VTE prophylaxis.

Tips

- More blood loss may occur postoperatively than intraoperatively.
- Patients will be taught "hip precautions"—avoidance of flexion/rotation, avoidance of deep flexion, and others—to minimize the likelihood of dislocation of the hip prosthesis.
- Patients who have undergone minimally invasive approach may go home on POD 1–2.
- Most primary (first-time) THAs are WBAT, but many revision THAs will be partial or protected weight bearing.

Common Issues to TKAs and THAs

- Both depression and use of narcotics prior to joint replacement are associated with clinical dissatisfaction after surgery. Consider minimizing narcotics to lowest tolerable dose in advance of elective surgery and working to assure depression is reasonably controlled.
- Patients with comorbidities, complications, or persistent drainage may have longer hospital courses.
- Revisions typically are more complex, take longer, and have more intraoperative blood loss.
- Hypotension is common on the night of surgery (POD 0), especially if insufficient volume is given intraoperatively or if indwelling epidural catheters are used; IV fluid boluses in appropriate patients typically support patients through this.

For this reason, it is particularly important to write holding parameters for antihypertensive medications.

- Avoid 1/2 normal saline for IVF maintenance immediately postoperatively, which may contribute to hyponatremia in a patient who is slightly under-resuscitated; rather, normal saline or Lactated Ringers are appropriate.
- Commonly used drains include hemovac (round cylinder, uses springs to provide suction) and autovac (hemovac autotransfusion system—filters and reinfuses drained blood).
- Prophylactic antibiotics should be discontinued by 24 h postoperatively, unless otherwise indicated.
- Some centers use multimodal analgesic approaches (including long-acting oral analgesics, NSAIDs, and prophylactic antiemetics); use caution when introducing new medications, especially long-acting narcotics, in narcotic-naïve and older patients.
- Deep vein thrombosis (DVT) prophylaxis is typically the surgeon's choice, though good to engage in conversation with surgeons if the patient's risk for DVT deviates from the norm. Know that there are differences between the American Academy of Orthopedic Surgeons (AAOS) and American College of Chest Physicians (ACCP) guidelines. Common agents are low-molecular-weight heparins, warfarin, and aspirin (in addition to TEDs and SCDs).
- Be aware of hip precautions when examining patients—they may be prohibited from crossing legs initially. Check with the orthopedic surgeon if you need to move the patient for an examination.

HIP FRACTURE REPAIR
1–3 h/GA or regional/EBL 300 mL.

Tips
- There are various options for operative repair, including intramedullary nail, dynamic hip screw, and hemi- or total arthroplasty.
- Preoperative evaluation should include cardiovascular risk stratification, assessment for the presence of medical factors contributing to fracture (e.g., seizure or syncope), and recommendations for perioperative medication management.
- Surgery should not be delayed for minor medical conditions (e.g., poorly controlled hypertension without hypertensive urgency or emergency).
- If surgery is to be delayed, VTE prophylaxis should be encouraged, as there is risk of VTE from the fracture itself even without surgery.

TOTAL SHOULDER ARTHROPLASTY

3 h/GA (occasionally regional), EBL < 500 mL.

POD 0: Advance diet. Stop IV fluids if doing well with oral intake. PCA for initial pain control, with transition to oral medications the evening of surgery. Continuous passive motion (CPM) machine commonly used.

POD 1: Drain out. Continued physical therapy, CPM machine.

POD 2: Discharge to home.

Tips

- Pharmacologic VTE prophylaxis is not used if patients are ambulating.
- Postoperative bleeding/hemarthrosis is not uncommon after total shoulder arthroplasty (TSA). In patients who are on therapeutic anticoagulation (for atrial fibrillation, heart valve, history of VTE, others), work closely with the patient's surgeon and primary cardiologist (if applicable) to determine the best time to resume therapeutic anticoagulation. Ideally, avoid anticoagulation in the first several days postoperatively unless the risk of clot is exceedingly high (e.g., mitral valve prosthesis).
- If a scalene block is used, adverse effects include hypotension, bradycardia, Horner's syndrome, and phrenic nerve involvement, causing diaphragmatic paralysis and sudden onset of pain late in the night or early morning as block wears off.

MAJOR SPINE SURGERY

10+ h/GA/EBL 3,000+ mL.

POD 0: ICU care until stabilized. Remain intubated for airway protection and pain control. Often require additional transfusions.

POD 1–2: Extubate when stable; transfer to floor.

POD 3–7: VTE prophylaxis when possible; mobilization using brace, drain care.

Tips

- These are high-risk operations due to their blood loss and duration.
- EBL can reach as much as 10 L.
- Often operations are accomplished in 2–3 stages.
- Patients are at risk for multiple complications including venous thromboembolic events (VTE), myocardial infarction,

pneumonia, disseminated intravascular coagulation, dilutional coagulopathy, posterior ischemic optic neuropathy (blindness—rare, but devastating), dural leak, cerebrospinal fluid leak (may be difficult to detect), hematoma, secondary meningitis (can be subtle—may present with confusion, low-grade fever, headache), facial/airway edema from prone position, and ileus.

- Occasionally patients receive pulse-dose steroids.
- Rehab/skilled nursing facility is a common disposition.
- Spine precautions—patients commonly require a brace.

OTHER SPINE SURGERY

Lumbar spine decompressions/fusions are of intermediate risk, typically involve a 3–4-day hospital stay, and patients are admitted directly to the floor.

- C-spine decompressions often have a shorter stay, e.g., 24–48 h.
- Microdecompressions are typically limited-stay procedures.

ORTHOPEDIC TUMOR SURGERY

4+ h/GA/EBL highly variable.

Complex and varied. Range from peripheral tumors to combined procedures with general surgery and urology in the pelvic and abdominal cavity. Many have long duration, high EBL, and long length of stay, similar to major spine operations.

Tips

- Generally intermediate-risk operations, but can be of high risk depending on duration and blood loss.
- Tumors are often highly vascular, contributing to higher EBLs and drain output.
- Sudden increase in drain output after pelvic surgery may be a sign of ureter disruption.
- Surgery service may be reluctant to initiate heparin-based VTE prophylaxis due to wound drainage—discuss with primary team.

GENERAL SURGERY

For bariatric procedures, see also Chap. 38.

GASTRIC BYPASS, LAPAROSCOPIC

2.5–3.5 h/GA/EBL 50–200 mL.

POD 0: ICU or step-down unit for patients with OSA.

POD 1: Start bariatric clear liquid diet and ADAT to full liquids/pureed. Start oral medications (crushed/liquid only for 2 weeks). Transfer to floor (if needed ICU post-op). Urinary catheter removed.

POD 2: PT/OT clearance, registered dietician (RD) teaching. Discharge home.

GASTRIC BYPASS, OPEN
2.5–3.5 h/GA/EBL 100–400 mL (varies).

POD 0: ICU or other close respiratory monitoring for patients with OSA.

POD 1: Start bariatric clear liquid diet and ADAT to full liquids/pureed. Start oral medications (crushed or liquid only for 2 weeks). Transfer to floor (if needed ICU post-op). Urinary catheter removed.

POD 2–3: Remove epidural. Transition to oral pain medications.

POD 4: Discharge home.

SLEEVE GASTRECTOMY
1–2 h/GA/EBL 50–100 mL.

POD 0: ICU or step-down unit for patients with OSA.

POD 1: Start bariatric clear liquid diet and ADAT to full liquids/pureed. Start oral medications (crushed or liquid only for 2 weeks). Discharge home in the afternoon/evening.

LAPAROSCOPIC BAND
1 h/GA/EBL minimal.

POD 0: Limited stay. Start bariatric clear liquid diet and ADAT to full liquids/pureed. Start oral medications (crushed or liquid only for 2 weeks).

POD 1: Discharge home.

ESOPHAGECTOMY
6 h/GA + epidural/EBL varies.

POD 0: ICU. May have chest tubes.

POD 1–5: Mobilize; transfer to floor when possible. Strictly NPO until passes UGI series POD 5 or later. Usually not on TPN unless remains NPO past POD 5.

Tips

- Complications can be serious, including acute respiratory distress syndrome (ARDS), pericarditis, pneumothorax, pneumonia, and anastomotic leak. In our experience with the patients of higher medical risk, ICU stays are several days.
- Widened mediastinum on CXR may be due to postoperative changes; anastomosis may be at stomach vs. jejunum.
- Most patients have some degree of chest pain post-op due to the location of the surgery.
- Transhiatal approach involves an abdominal incision and a left neck incision. Proximity to heart and great vessels may cause intraoperative hypotension and arrhythmias.
- Post-op atrial fibrillation is very common; one of the main difficulties in treating it is the prolonged NPO status.
- Do not use CPAP initially after esophagectomy.
- Do not reposition or move NG tube.

HERNIA REPAIR

Varies greatly from outpatient inguinal hernia repair under local anesthesia to major abdominal operation. Note that some lung diseases, e.g., severe COPD, may be worsened with repair of a ventral hernia due to increased intra-abdominal pressure.

WHIPPLE (PANCREATICODUODENECTOMY)

8–12 h/GA + epidural/EBL 500–1,000 mL.

Tips

- Usually prolonged postoperative course, initially in ICU, with prolonged return of bowel function.
- Often J tubes are placed for enteral nutrition.
- Increased drain output may be from chylous, pancreatic, or biliary leak.
- Some patients develop insulin-dependent DM postoperatively, depending on the extent of the pancreatic resection.
- If a patient returns from surgery very quickly, it likely means that there was unresectable disease and no further operation was performed. Always wait for the surgeon to discuss this with the patient.
- Complications include line infection, pneumonia, ARDS, portal vein thrombosis, and lateral cutaneous nerve injury from retractors.

LIVER RESECTION
6 h/GA + epidural/EBL variable.

Tips

- Extent of resection varies; often patients are very ill at baseline due to underlying liver disease.
- ICU post-op can have high EBL, hepatic dysfunction, ARDS.

GYNECOLOGY AND GYNECOLOGY–ONCOLOGY SURGERY

LAPAROSCOPIC TOTAL ABDOMINAL HYSTERECTOMY–BILATERAL SALPINGO-OOPHORECTOMY: ROBOT ASSIST OR CONVENTIONAL
1–3 h/GA/EBL < 100 mL.

POD 0: Can advance diet if no nausea/vomiting post-op.

POD 1: Diet advanced; PO pain medications; urinary catheter out and discharge.

Tips

- An increasing percentage of hysterectomies are now done robotically. For laparoscopic or robotic, patients may have shoulder pain from gas under the diaphragm, but they are able to ambulate and have earlier return of bowel function than with a total abdominal hysterectomy–bilateral salpingo-oophorectomy (TAH–BSO).
- Some patients are discharged on the same day as surgery.
- Some obese patients may actually require an overnight ICU stay due to prolonged Trendelenburg positioning.

VAGINAL HYSTERECTOMY WITH PELVIC ORGAN PROLAPSE REPAIR (E.G., ANTERIOR AND POSTERIOR REPAIR, VAGINAL VAULT SUSPENSION, SLING FOR URINARY INCONTINENCE)
2–3 h/GA or regional/EBL < 200 mL.

POD 0: Advance diet if tolerated.

POD 1: Diet advanced; change to PO pain medications. Voiding trial done with checking of post-void residual volume.

Tips
- Only about 1/3 of women void adequately on POD 1 after complex vaginal repairs. 2/3 go home with a catheter.

OPEN TAH–BSO (FOR BENIGN PATHOLOGY)
2 h/GA/EBL 100 mL.

POD 0: If there has been an intestinal anastomosis, then NPO until flatus; otherwise diet advanced.

POD 1–2: Diet advanced as above, urinary catheter out, change to PO pain meds.

POD 2–3: Discharge to home.

Tips
- Rarely done given rising prevalence of laparoscopic and robotic surgeries.
- These procedures tend to have earlier return of bowel function than general surgery cases that involve more of the GI tract, but later than minimally invasive procedures.

OPEN TAH–BSO (FOR MALIGNANCY)
2–4 h/GA/EBL 100–1,000 mL.

POD 0: If there has been an intestinal anastomosis, then NPO until flatus; otherwise diet advanced.

POD 1–2: Diet advanced as above; urinary catheter out; change to PO pain meds.

POD 3: Discharge to home.

Tips
- In some cases, it is unknown whether the tumor is benign or malignant preoperatively.
- Depending on tumor burden, this operation may be longer and involve bowel resection, lymph node dissection, and/or omentectomy, with a higher EBL and longer duration. There may be delayed return of bowel function as a result.
- Depending on the type of hysterectomy, there may be a need for prolonged urinary catheterization.
- If malignancy, there is increased VTE risk, so VTE prophylaxis is often continued after discharge.

OVARIAN TUMOR DEBULKING OR CYTOREDUCTION (PELVIC EXENTERATION RARELY DONE)

7–10+ h/GA + epidural/EBL 1,000+ mL.

Often in the hospital 7–14 days.

Tips

- Patients with advanced ovarian cancer may have significant ascites and/or electrolyte abnormalities.
- Exenteration typically results in ileostomy/colostomy and urostomy.
- Patients are often observed in ICU postoperatively.
- Expect extensive blood loss and fluid shifts requiring additional resuscitation.
- May have prolonged ileus requiring parenteral nutrition.
- Complications include sepsis/ARDS, urinoma/ureter disruption, VTE, pelvic abscess, as well as atrial fibrillation on POD 2–3.

UROLOGIC SURGERY/ PROCEDURES

CYSTECTOMY, RADICAL

Removal of the bladder and prostate in men; removal of the bladder, possibly uterus and ovaries, possibly anterior vaginal strip in women. Urinary diversion with ileal conduit, neobladder to the urethra, or cutaneous neobladder to the abdominal wall.

6+ h (varies, longer for robotic)/GA + epidural/EBL 500–1,500 (varies).

POD 0: NPO.

POD 1–3: NPO, follow drain output; some urologists give early clears, regular diet POD 2.

POD 4–5: Bowel function usually returns.

Tips

- Generally no per rectum (PR) meds initially.
- Delayed postoperative ileus often occurs (and may last a week or more), even after apparent return of bowel function.
- High risk for VTE events, patients discharge with a month of low-molecular-weight heparin (LMWH) prophylaxis.

PROSTATECTOMY, RADICAL
2–5 h/GA/EBL 200–1,000 mL.

Typical length of stay is 1–2 days for robotic or open.

Tips
- Main issue is attention to blood loss; this is less of an issue now that many are done robotically.

TRANSURETHRAL RESECTION OF PROSTATE
1 h or less/GA or spinal/EBL minimal to 300 mL (varies, hard to quantify).

Many go home on the same day, especially if they had a GreenLight laser TURP.

Tips
- Watch for obstructing clots, problematic on continuous bladder irrigation

NEPHRECTOMY WITH INFERIOR VENA CAVA THROMBECTOMY
4–8 h (depending on the height of the thrombus)/GA + epidural/EBL varies, often >1 L.

Often require ICU care postoperatively (unless thrombus is small).

Liver surgeon may assist if there is need for mobilization of the liver.

Thoracic surgeon may perform part of the thrombectomy via sternotomy if thrombus extends above the diaphragm. Intraoperative concern for emboli from manipulation of IVC thrombus.

Tips
- Watch for pneumothorax, pleural effusion, hemothorax, hepatic dysfunction, sequela of intraoperative emboli from manipulation of thrombus, and ileus; also, other ICU complications such as pneumonia, catheter-associated infections, etc.
- Often greater bowel manipulation than radical nephrectomy without thrombectomy
- High risk for VTE events, patients may discharge with a month of LMWH prophylaxis

OPEN NEPHRECTOMY, RADICAL
3–4 h/GA + epidural/300 mL.

POD 1–3 advance diet when bowel function returns.

Tips
- Anticipate increased creatinine/renal dosing of medications.
- Diet can usually be advanced expeditiously, if bowel is not manipulated.

LAPAROSCOPIC NEPHRECTOMY

4 h/GA/100 mL.

POD 0—Diet may be advanced.

In some cases, patients may be discharged on POD 1.

Tips

- Anticipate increased creatinine/renal dosing of medications.

OPEN PARTIAL NEPHRECTOMY

3–4 h/GA + epidural/300 mL.

POD 1–3 advance diet when bowel function returns.

Tips

- Usually no increased creatinine or need for renal dosing of medications; look for other causes, if kidney injury develops
- Main issues are bleeding and urinary leak: Usually on bed rest for 24–48 h with drain in place

LAPAROSCOPIC/ROBOTIC PARTIAL NEPHRECTOMY

4–6 h/GA/100 mL.

POD 0—Diet may be advanced.

In some cases, patients may be discharged on POD 1.

Tips

- Almost always stay 2–3 days for drain/urinary catheter management and observation for bleeding.
- Usually no increased creatinine or need for renal dosing of medications (look for other causes).
- Main issues are bleeding and urinary leak: Usually on bed rest for 24–48 h with drain in place.

CYSTOSCOPY, TRANSURETHRAL RESECTION OF BLADDER TUMOR (TURBT), LITHOTRIPSY

Duration varies/moderate sedation vs. GA/EBL varies.

These are typically outpatient or limited-stay procedures.

Tips

- Note that cystoscopy may have risk of increased vagal tone, bradycardia, and hypotension, despite being considered a low-risk procedure.

VASCULAR SURGERY

GENERAL CONSIDERATIONS
■ Continue preoperative beta-blockade in the postoperative setting.
■ Decisions about anticoagulants and antiplatelet agents are made at the discretion of the surgeon based on the magnitude of the procedure and the patients individualized risk of thrombotic and/or bleeding complications. Many patients undergoing vascular surgical procedures should continue their aspirin perioperatively but this should be discussed with the surgeon.
■ Statins are associated with reduction in cardiovascular events and thought to play a beneficial role in atherosclerotic plaque stability and possibly rate of aneurysm degeneration. As such, most vascular surgery patients should be on a statin unless specifically contraindicated.

CAROTID ENDARTERECTOMY (CEA)
3–4 h/GA/150 mL.

POD 0: ICU.

POD 1: Remove urinary catheter, advance diet. Transfer to floor. Possible D/C home.

POD 2: Discharge to home.

Tips
■ Procedure carries risk of myocardial infarction, stroke, and cranial nerve injury.
■ Postoperative blood pressure control can require IV medications as endarterectomy can alter function of the baroreceptor in the carotid sinus.
■ Needs postoperative blood pressure control and close neurologic examinations.

ABDOMINAL AORTIC ANEURYSM REPAIR, OPEN
6 h/GA/EBL 400–1,000 mL.

POD 0: ICU. May come out of OR still intubated.

POD 1–3: Stabilize, transfer to floor.

POD 4–6: Epidural out, then urinary catheter out.

Tips

- Variation in length of ICU stay.
- Level of proximal aortic cross clamp predicts morbidity of the operation. Infrarenal is least stressful, suprarenal is more stressful, and supravisceral (aka supraceliac) is most stressful.
- Nonoliguric acute renal failure can occur with suprarenal cross-clamping of the aorta. Reviewing the operative note is helpful.
- Other severe complications include bowel infarction and spinal cord infarct.

AAA REPAIR, ENDOVASCULAR
3 h/GA/EBL 50–200 mL.

POD 0: ICU. Short post-op hydration for IV contrast load, but rarely require resuscitation.

POD 1: Urinary catheter out in AM. Check renal function. Regular diet. Often go home.

Tips

- Much lower level of overall physiologic stress than open repair, therefore less time in ICU and shorter overall hospital course.
- Patients require lifelong follow-up after discharge for monitoring for stent migration or endoleak; usually CT at 1 month, then at 6–12 months, and annually thereafter (but imaging schedule may differ per surgeon).
- Severe complications include groin hematoma, endoleak, kidney injury from embolization or contrast, bowel ischemia, and spinal cord infarct (rare).

PERIPHERAL VASCULAR DISEASE BYPASS, SUPRAINGUINAL
4–6 h/GA/EBL 250–1,000 mL.

POD 0: ICU. May come out of OR intubated. Resuscitation.

POD 1–2: Stabilize, wean resuscitation by 48 h. To floor.

POD 3–5: Resume diet. Epidural and urinary catheter out. Walking.

Tips

- Similar to open abdominal aortic aneurysm (AAA) repair, but usually reserved for healthier patients with peripheral vascular disease (PVD). Clamp is most often below the renal arteries, so typically better tolerated than AAA repair.

PVD BYPASS, INFRAINGUINAL
4–5 h/GA/EBL 200–400 mL.

POD 0: ICU for pulse checks. Do not need resuscitation.

POD 1–3: Floor. Wound care. Urinary catheter out.

Tips
- Length of stay is often a function of mobility status and foot wounds/ulcerations.

HEAD AND NECK SURGERY

TRACHEOTOMY (NEW)
15–30 min/typically GA, can be done under local anesthesia/EBL minimal.

POD 0: ICU or other specialized ward for airway monitoring.

POD 1: May be transferred to floor if doing well.

Tips
- May be straightforward or complex depending on the patient's anatomy and previous operations, if any.
- Common early complications are obstruction or displacement of the tracheostomy tube.
- If acute airway obstruction is suspected, the inner cannula of the tracheostomy tube may be removed. Also, direct suctioning through the tracheostomy tube can alleviate mucus plugging that can cause obstruction.

HEAD AND NECK CANCER RESECTION/MICROVASCULAR FREE FLAP/LARYNGECTOMY
8+ h/GA/EBL variable.

Tips
- Can be extensive operations of long duration, although fluid shifts are typically minimal given the location.
- Most patients are in the ICU initially if a new tracheotomy is involved or a microvascular free flap is placed.
- Free flaps are commonly harvested from the forearm, lower leg (fibula), and thigh. Flaps may also be harvested from the chest, abdomen, or back. You may see drains in multiple sites.

- Free flap patients are often started on aspirin POD#1 to optimize blood flow through flap, but re-initiation of anticoagulation may be delayed longer dependent on comfort of surgical team.
- For patients undergoing resection and reconstruction of the oral cavity or pharynx, nutrition is commonly initially provided via a nasogastric tube to avoid damage to the oral cavity or pharyngeal reconstruction. If the patient is at high risk of prolonged dysphagia from the procedure, a gastrostomy tube maybe placed.
- Laryngectomy patients are typically not permitted oral intake for a week postoperatively and are either fed through a nasogastric tube, gastrostomy tube, or potentially a tracheoesophageal catheter placed intraoperatively.
- Laryngectomy patients have the safest airway possible.
- Communication may be difficult with patients due to alteration of anatomy.
- Alcohol withdrawal and COPD are common given the patient population's comorbid risk factors.
- Overall hospital stay is approximately 7 days.

HEAD AND NECK DISSECTION
2–4 h/GA/EBL minimal.

Tips

- Can be an extensive operation of long duration, although fluid shifts are typically minimal given the location.
- May be admitted to the floor if shorter duration of operation and no tracheostomy.
- A drain may be placed in the neck.
- Hospital stay is typically 2–3 days.
- Alcohol withdrawal and COPD are common given the patient population's comorbid risk factors.

NEUROSURGERY

CRANIOTOMY
6–24 h/GA/EBL variable.

Tips

- Variable course, depending on the extent of surgery and condition necessitating surgery.

- Initially admitted to ICU, may have ICP monitor, often still intubated.
- First few days post-op may have labile blood pressures and hyponatremia. Neurosurgery team will often administer mannitol and salt tabs and order serial CT scans.
- Watch for ICU complications such as VTE, line infections, and PNA.
- May have a great deal of facial swelling post-op.

VENTRICULOPERITONEAL (VP) SHUNT
1–2 h/GA/EBL 5–10 mL.

Tips
- Often admitted to ICU for frequent neuro checks for the first 24 h post-op
- In hospital for 1–3 days for pain control, return of bowel function
- Watch for ileus, surgical site infection, and spinal headache

ENDOVASCULAR ANEURYSM COILING
Duration varies by complexity/GA/minimal EBL.

Tips
- Know the surgical plan—this is often a precursor to open clipping.
- Often a 24-h admission for hourly neuro checks then home.
- Watch for hypertension, new neuro findings.
- Neurosurgeons may monitor for vasospasm with transcranial dopplers.

OPHTHALMOLOGIC SURGERY

CATARACT SURGERY
2–3 h/GA or local/EBL minute.

Usually an outpatient procedure. A widely cited study (N Engl J Med 2000;342:168–75) randomized patients to ECG and lab tests vs. no standard preoperative tests and found no difference in complication rates. However, all patients did receive a pre-op H&P. We advocate an evaluation by a primary care provider and lab testing only as indicated preoperatively. Warfarin anticoagulation typically does not have to be held as long as the INR < 3.0, but it is best to check with the surgeon. Note also that tamsulosin has been associated with "intraoperative floppy iris syndrome" and should be held for 2 weeks pre-op.

DENTAL SURGERY

Preoperative evaluation for patients with multiple medical comorbidities who are to undergo general anesthesia for dental extractions should focus on a complete H&P and ensure that there is no active or decompensated medical problems. Patients on warfarin may be able to remain on anticoagulation as long as the INR is <3.0 and there is no greater than average bleeding risk for the surgery.

Index

M.B. Jackson et al. (eds.), *The Perioperative Medicine Consult Handbook*, DOI 10.1007/978-3-319-09366-6,
© Springer International Publishing Switzerland 2015

Made in the USA
Middletown, DE
21 September 2015